DATE DUE

DE ~~3 02~~			
DE 17 05			

DEMCO 38-296

THE TOTAL GUIDE
TO A
HEALTHY HEART

THE TOTAL GUIDE TO A HEALTHY HEART

INTEGRATIVE STRATEGIES FOR PREVENTING AND REVERSING HEART DISEASE

SETH J. BAUM, M.D., F.A.C.C.

Kensington Books
http://www.kensingtonbooks.com

...accurate and authoritative in-
...ct matter covered. It is sold
with the understanding that the publisher is not engaged in
rendering medical or related professional services and that
without personal consultation the author cannot and does not
render judgment or advice about a particular patient or medical condition. If medical advice is required, the services of a
competent professional should be sought. While every attempt has been made to provide accurate information, the author and publisher cannot be held responsible for any errors
or omissions.

KENSINGTON BOOKS are published by

Kensington Publishing Corp.
850 Third Avenue
New York, NY 10022

Library of Congress Card Catalogue Number: 98-075687
ISBN 1-57566-448-8

First Printing: September, 1999
10 9 8 7 6 5 4 3 2 1

With eternal love, gratitude, and appreciation, I dedicate this book to my wife, Laura, and our three children, Jason, Jared, and Kyra—my guiding lights and the firm foundation without whom I could neither weather the storms of life nor fully feel the warmest rays of sunshine.

Acknowledgments

To all the wonderful people who helped make this book possible, thank you:

- Vicki Accardi, my agent and friend, for her "behind the scenes" vitality and tenacity.
- Andrea Peralta, my transcriptionist who, at the drop of a hat, would re-rewrite sections of this book (even on weekends).
- Larry Sugar and Jolie Root, for guiding me through the early days of my education about natural remedies.
- John and Susan Carlson, who have supported many of my seminars at which I've been able to spread the word about the evolving field of integrative cardiology.
- Liz Wertman, Elaine Barone, and Diane Korber, my office staff, who patiently accepted my harried and oftentimes chaotic existence during the creation of this book.
- Allan Graubard, Paul Dinas and Walter Zacharius, for their involvement with the book.
- Lee Heiman, for his keen comprehension of the alternative medicine world.
- Tracy Bernstein, for being accessible and dependable, but most important, extremely funny.
- Neenyah Ostram, my editorial consultant, whose skill with charts helped bring my book to life.
- Nancy Szeman, for her nutritional expertise and her whole-hearted dedication to our center.
- Joan Andres, for her knowledge of stress and ways to reduce it.
- Shaun O'Hare, for his great expertise in the area of physical fitness, and his patience while "whipping" me into shape.
- Nancy Ash, for bringing her yoga skills to our center.
- Rina Vinci, for her talent and gift with Reiki, and for helping me to understand firsthand the power of Energy.

- Arthur Rosenfeld, for his dynamic and brilliant T'ai Chi teaching skills (and his non–T'ai Chi brilliance, as well).
- Dr. Robert Willix, for being brave enough to have taken the path he did and kind enough to let me share his story with you.
- The St. Jude Medical Company, for generously allowing me to reprint their excellent pictures of heart valves.
- Jodi Zheutlin, who gave me an honest appraisal of the book in its early stages.
- Dr. Helen Barold, for her "woman's perspective" of electrophysiology.
- Dr. David Rubin, my mentor and friend.
- Drs. Melvin Weiss and Martin Cohen, for training me in angioplasty.
- Drs. Carmine Sorbera, Anthony Pucillo, Richard Kay, Jeffrey Blake, Robert Belkin, Craig Munsen, for providing me with the opportunity to develop a firm foundation in cardiology.
- Dr. Joseph Pizzorno, whose publications and work at Bastyr University showed me the science behind natural medicine.
- Stanley and Joyce Prieser, for being great friends and advisors.
- My son Jason, for his computer expertise.
- My parents, Morton and Elissa, and siblings, Simeon and Debbie, "for just being there."
- My wife's parents, Bruce and Delia Denson, for raising such a wonderful woman.
- Betty Paris, for entertaining my children during my too-frequent absences.
- My dog, Beau, for frequently awakening me at 3 A.M. and thereby providing me with a quiet and creative time to do some of my best writing.

Contents

Introduction xi

Chapter 1
The Birth of Integrative Heart Care 1

Chapter 2
The Heart in Harmony 9

Chapter 3
Heart Tests: Understanding Them Will Dissolve Your Fears 17

Chapter 4
Heart Breakers: The Many Causes of Coronary Disease 33

Chapter 5
The Pipes Are Clogged 63

Chapter 6
Call 911—It's "The Big One" 87

Chapter 7
Heart Failure: When the Muscle Doesn't Squeeze 103

Chapter 8
Valvular Heart Disease: Disorders of "Too Much" and "Too Little" 121

Chapter 9
Electrophysiology: The Shocking Truth 139

Chapter 10
If Chicken Soup Is Penicillin, Then What Is This I'm Eating? 151

Chapter 11
How the Health Food Store Can Help Your Heart 171

Chapter 12
  Nature's Edible Gifts 195

Chapter 13
  To Sweat or Not to Sweat—It Is No Longer a Question 215

Chapter 14
  You Needn't Be a Yogi to Be Relaxed 223

Chapter 15
  The Future of Integrative Heart Care 235

Suggested Reading 241

Glossary 245

Appendix
  Abnormal Heart Rhythms and Their Treatments 253

Generic and Trade Name Drugs 271

Bibliography 275

Resource Guide 279

Index 289

Introduction

Modern medicine is magical. Walk through an operating suite and you can witness wonders. See the man whose heart stopped during the throes of a heart attack restarted in an emergency room, prior to its being restopped and restarted during a bypass operation, ultimately adding countless years to his life. Observe the blind father undergoing a corneal transplant: The surgeon carefully removes the cornea from a recently deceased person and then meticulously sews it onto the blind man's eye, restoring his visual connection to his family and all life around him. Watch the young child being whisked into the trauma suite to have his severed limb reattached so he can live a normal and unencumbered existence. Medicine's list of miracles is nearly interminable. Modern medicine is truly transcendent. Why, then, search for something better? How is medicine flawed?

The frailty of medicine lies in its very strength, its "modernity." Modern medicine is impatient. To be satisfied and successful, modern physicians must achieve the ultimate quick-fix. As you can see, in many circumstances, physicians have been able to do this. The speedy solution, although essential in many situations, is not always the complete solution. To cure medicine of its deficiencies, we—physicians and patients alike—must learn patience. We require patience in healing, in being healed, and in preventing illness.

By reflecting on the lessons of ancient healers, who understood the value of patience in achieving health, we *can* find a way to a more balanced practice for health. A central theme in the ancient arts of Ayurveda and Chinese medicine, as well as in the ancient

Judeo-Christian forms of healing, is the unity of mind and body. Existing not in isolation, but intimately and indistinguishably intertwined, mind and body must each be healthy for the other to be free of illness. To treat an illness in one is to treat an illness in the other. The ancient physician's approach to the ailing patient was slow and steady. It focused as much on teaching patients how to influence their own bodies as what to take from nature to help them to do so. Through meditation and self-exploration, for example, patients were taught to reduce stress, achieve improved inner tranquillity, and gain greater health. Of course, lacking modern technological advances, ancient physicians were unable to avert the immediate, acute tragedies that I and other physicians treat so adroitly today. Ancient physicians, however, used other gifts, the gifts they found in nature as their armamentarium.

Herbs, for instance, were a frequently used means of healing in all ancient forms of medicine. And while we may initially scoff at the possibility that plants can possess profound medicinal qualities, in fact we continue to use herbs in medicine today—with herbs constituting the basis for nearly 25–30 percent of all medicines prescribed in America.

Another "gift of nature" utilized so effectively by the ancients lies within each of us: the ability to heal ourselves through meditation and self-understanding. Unfortunately, being "modern and scientific," we often cringe at the suggestion of deeper and more philosophical possibilities. We must overcome our modernization to become healthier. By examining and understanding what the ancient physicians taught, we can complete and thus cure our own medical system.

Thus, I call for a marriage of the old and the new. With the union of modern medicine and ancient medical wisdom, not only can we cure dramatic, acute illness, but also aid the chronically ill and, in many cases, help to prevent acute illness from developing in the first place. As a cardiologist trained in the most modern, cutting-edge procedures, such as angioplasties, rotoblators, and stents, I understand the need for technology-based medicine. I also appreciate modern medicine's boundaries and limitations. I understand that taking a patient through a life-saving bypass operation, although wonderful, is incomplete. We need to explore and correct those factors that precipitated this patient's heart problem to prevent him or her from returning for a future, repeat operation. In fact, I would like to prevent my patients, and patients everywhere, from ever developing heart disease, from ever needing to become a "patient" at all. But to do so, a balanced harmony of old and new forms of medicine is necessary.

I have begun to achieve this kind of harmony in my own cardiology practice. With the help of such men as Dr. Andrew Weil, Dr. Dean Ornich, and Dr. Isadore Rosenfeld, I have been able to open my mind to the vast world of "alternative possibilities."

In this book, then, I will help you to understand how the heart functions in both health and disease. Together, we will explore the heart tests doctors use, what we've learned about heart disease, and what we can do to prevent it. By developing a thorough understanding of the heart, we will all become more educated "health consumers."

As I take you through the world of the heart, all the while broadening our sense of the great possibilities that heart medicine possesses, I do so with this memory as well. I recall my first days of learning (and subsequently teaching) the martial arts discipline of Tae Kwon Do. Watching the black belts fly through the air, spinning, kicking and fracturing boards with keen and controlled accuracy, I yearned for the time when I, too, could perform such techniques. Before ever throwing my first kick, however, I spent an entire year mastering the basics of stances, blocks, and punches. When I finally reached the point at which I was ready to learn the marvelous moves I'd so admired, I understood the significance of patience, of my basic training. My task was made infinitely easier and my development dramatically enhanced because of my prior efforts to create a strong foundation on which to build.

So it is with the heart, yours and mine. We must first understand how the heart works before we can safely and appropriately incorporate into our lives the many miraculous life-promoting, heart-enhancing natural solutions now available to us all. And this is what I will share with you in *The Total Guide to a Healthy Heart*. In the integration of modern and ancient forms of medicine, we will find the balance we so desperately need, both patients and physicians alike. And as we do so, we will create the kind of health care system we wish to have, responsive to our needs and offering possibilities of cure and care that we simply cannot do without.

The Birth of Integrative Heart Care

I am an interventional cardiologist. My title betrays me. As an "intervener"—a specialized warrior in the battle against heart disease—I have snaked catheters, wires, balloons, lasers, and drills into the arteries of thousands of patients to prevent or minimize heart attacks. I feel blessed to have had such a personal and dramatic impact on the lives of so many people. Over the years, however, I have seen numerous patients return, requiring repeats of procedures such as bypass grafting and angioplasty. Frustrated by the apparent failures of the cutting-edge techniques available to me, I have also felt my patients' frustration. As you will learn though, our frustration levels have diminished through the successful practice of a more integrated form of medicine.

Be that as it may, some people, instead of acknowledging that modern ("allopathic") medicine has its strengths and weaknesses, completely discard traditional medical approaches. At times, patients refuse to undergo angioplasties because of the prior negative experiences of friends or relatives. Sadly, too, some people sacrifice their lives when refusing these procedures. I know this all too well. I have helplessly observed patients die as they rejected the life-saving procedures of allopathic medicine.

Through my involvement in the lives and deaths of people I have treated, I have found myself torn apart by the same contradictions and questions that plague many of us today. If modern cardiology is perfect, then why do so many people need second and third bypasses or angioplasties? Sure, modern medicine saves lives, but by doing little to treat underlying disease, it often condemns patients to return for repeat procedures. I, too, have sometimes wondered whether allopathic medicine should be abandoned altogether in favor of a more natural approach to healing. If nothing else, this would enable patients and healers to relate more humanly and intimately than they do now.

After years of self-examination, however, I no longer expect perfection from either modern or alternative medicine. Both clearly possess strengths and weaknesses. Simplistically stated, modern medicine treats immediate, life-threatening conditions while alternative medicine addresses more chronic problems. I also know that the two forms must find common ground for healing to become a reality. So I dreamed of a new, integrated form of cardiology and yearned for the strength to begin practicing what I felt to be right. After all, as a physician, I am obligated—in fact, I am oath-bound—to explore any avenue that may benefit my patients, no matter how foreign the route may be.

As my personal exploration began, I devoured thousands of pages of data regarding natural remedies for heart disease. In fact, my endeavor was so intense that I often felt I was back in medical school, burning the candle at both ends simply to become fluent in the new, majestic language of "natural medicine." As my knowledge of vitamins, minerals, herbs, and other natural supplements blossomed, so too did my certainty that I was following a worthy path. I was ready to make the leap into practicing integrative medicine.

And so I did. Mr. Joseph Goldberg, an affable, intelligent, and physically fit 65-year-old man, had suffered from high blood pressure and high cholesterol for years. Understanding the importance of exercise, he played tennis three to five times a week without any difficulty. Over the past several months, however, he had developed a disturbing pressure in his chest whenever he played tennis. Within the past two to three weeks, he also noted that he would suffer from this discomfort when walking, forcing him to discontinue even mild physical activity. This was devastating to Mr. Goldberg, for he not only appreciated the importance of exercise, he truly loved to be active.

Mr. Goldberg consulted his family doctor who, after performing a stress test, found him to need a cardiac catheterization (also called an angiogram). In this procedure, an invasive cardiologist (like me) punctures the artery in the groin and passes fine tubes into the arteries of the heart to define their anatomy. It is extremely rare to experience a complication during this exam, but 1 in 1,000 patients suffers from any number of complications, running the gamut from bleeding excessively to having a stroke or even dying. Although it is terrifying to undergo a procedure where death is a possibility, however remote, it is sometimes necessary to do so if only to achieve greater benefit. I agreed with Mr. Goldberg's family physician that our patient could benefit from the angiogram—that its risks were well warranted—and Mr. Goldberg consented.

The catheterization suite (where angiograms are performed) is an interesting place. There is an ambient levity that often seems inappropriate under such serious circumstances, but most patients enjoy the cheerfulness and lightness that the nursing and technical staff bring with them. The patient is brought into the suite lightly sedated. The nurses then place him on a hard, narrow, mobile table. Engulfed by a camera, TV monitor, and other essential equipment, he is otherwise naked. The nurses then place a "loin cloth" over his private parts (male patients often joke about the small size of their towel) and shave and cleanse the groin area with liquid soap. Subsequently, they cover him with a sterile drape. With the equipment set-up completed, the physician is called in.

This is how I found Mr. Goldberg upon entering the cath lab.

As Mr. Goldberg was experiencing the usual anxiety associated with an angiogram, he was given additional sedation. Only when he fell into near-sleep did I began the procedure. Lidocaine, a topical anesthetic, was injected into the groin area to numb it. A large needle was used to enter the femoral artery, easily recognizable by the forceful squirt of bright red blood shooting from the back of the needle once it's entered. A wire was then passed through the needle into the artery; the needle was removed and a sheath placed over the wire to rest within the center of the artery (the "lumen"). Once the wire was removed, we were ready for the catheters.

Catheters are long, fine tubes that pass through the arterial tree, back toward the heart. As catheters are hollow they allow us to measure pressure from the inside of the heart. We can also visualize the coronary arteries by injecting dye directly into them via the catheter. A large X-ray machine is used to take motion pictures of the arteries being filled by dye. Then we analyze the films to recommend further treatment options.

Mr. Goldberg's angiogram took about fifteen minutes. He was taken off the table, the tube was pulled from his groin, and pressure applied for twenty minutes to prevent any significant bleeding. He was to spend the next six hours lying still in bed so as not to disturb the nascent, delicate plug (i.e., scab) separating the inside of his artery from the rest of the world. Before sending Mr. Goldberg back to his room, I discussed the results of his procedure with him and his wife. All three of his arteries had significant disease—that is, blockage (atherosclerosis). His arteries, however, were not great candidates for either angioplasty or bypass; one artery was too small and the others possessed diffuse disease that covered a large area. On the positive side, his heart muscle was functioning well.

After considering the pros and cons of bypass, angioplasty, and medication, I advised bypass as a less than perfect but acceptable solution. They agreed. The whole discussion took about five minutes. Unbelievable—five minutes to make one of the most important decisions of a lifetime!

I left the room and felt, for the first time, a sick uneasiness about my decision to send Mr. Goldberg for heart surgery. Here was a patient who would not derive clear benefit from any particular approach in my allopathic armamentarium, yet I was trying to make him fit a mold which was not clearly his to fill. Within my "box" of traditional training, my choices were limited. The best that I could offer was a bypass. Yet I considered this as anything but a benign recommendation. He was about to undergo a procedure in which his chest would be sawed open; his heart would be stopped; and veins, stripped from his legs, would be reattached to the arteries that feed his heart. His risk of a serious complication (infection, stroke, or even death) would be 1–3 percent. And to make matters worse, the condition of his vessels, being poor candidates for surgery, indicated that he would have an incomplete and possibly short-lived result.

I left the hospital and agonized over this dilemma. My wife and I discussed it. I decided I would not let this be a five-minute decision. I would make my break from traditional medicine with Mr. Goldberg.

The following morning, I sat with Mr. and Mrs. Goldberg for an hour. We revisited the pros and cons of bypass surgery. I then described an alternative path, which combined stress reduction, nutritional counseling, exercise training, and herbal and vitamin therapy.

They chose the alternative route. I was thrilled. I was doing what I felt was right for my patient—not just in my mind, but in my heart. At that moment, I knew this was the proper path. I had a patient who wished to take responsibility for his own health care, and I would be there to help guide him in doing so.

I saw Mr. Goldberg in the office the following week—as I do all my post-catheterization patients—to check his groin, which was fine. However, this visit was different from all the other post-catheterization consultations I'd previously performed. Together, we spent a long time laying the groundwork for Mr. Goldberg's new form of treatment. I gave him a book on stress reduction. I outlined a graded exercise program we could follow based upon sound science, recognizing his specific needs and requirements, and enabling him to accelerate safely from walking to playing tennis free of angina. I prescribed vitamins and other nutritional supplements, including herbs to support his heart and help regulate his blood pressure. I sent him to my nutritionist, and scheduled a follow-up appointment in two weeks. Mr. Goldberg understood that he was to contact us with any problem or concern during that interval.

Two weeks later, he came to the office. The drop in his blood pressure astonished us both. Mr. Goldberg's blood pressure, which had run 160–180/90 for the past twenty to thirty years, was now 108/68. I checked and rechecked it. It didn't budge. It really was 108/68! After removing the childlike grin that covered my face, I reestablished myself as the cardiologist and shook his hand. Although I had acquired all the necessary intellectual tools for practicing a naturalist brand of cardiology, it was something altogether different to look squarely into the powerful face of nature. Here it was: Stress reduction, exercise, and natural supplements were accomplishing what an army of pharmaceuticals had failed to do.

Mr. Goldberg also generally felt better. He'd had only one episode of chest pain. He had lost several pounds and the chronic swelling in his feet had vanished. This was a great day for the Goldbergs, and for me as well. I stopped one of his blood pressure-lowering medicines, which he'd been taking for years, and made a follow-up appointment in another four weeks. Over these weeks, he was to have his blood pressure checked repeatedly to ensure its stability.

Well, Mr. Goldberg has since had many follow-up appointments.

His blood pressure has remained controlled, without traditional medicines. His cholesterol has dropped from 200 to 100 and I was thus able to withdraw his traditional (potentially toxic) cholesterol-lowering medications. He is fully active, back to tennis, and has had no more angina. In short, he feels great! In fact, he recently passed a stress test with flying colors—a sharp contrast to his failed test only a year and a half ago.

Mr. Goldberg is one of many such success stories. My patients are testimonials to the clear need for integrating allopathic and alternative forms of medicine. I still perform angioplasties and stents and still advise some of my patients to undergo bypass surgery. Fortunately, through the integration of natural therapies, I have been able to decrease the number of patients I now send for heart surgery. I also obtain a much more complete appraisal of my patients—although a cardiologist, I view my patients as whole beings, not just isolated hearts.

Although I make natural recommendations for all patients, neither I nor they consider them as panaceas. Many people still require operations to save their lives. Every patient is an individual; therefore, medical recommendations must be individualized. Now, of course, I think more about my medical decisions than I once did. I spend more time talking with my patients, and I offer them a wider range of therapeutic options to treat the underlying disease. I have begun practicing a form of cardiology that will become the standard in the twenty-first century.

As you're reading *The Total Guide to a Healthy Heart*, however, keep in mind this perspective; that although the numerous cardiovascular ailments you'll encounter are terrifying and at times require dramatic interventions, it remains my goal to *prevent* them *before* they strike. As I describe numerous natural approaches for preventing heart disease in the latter half of this book, I also wish at the outset to reinforce the absolute need for these practices to be integrated in all of our daily routines. I cannot begin to tell you how many of my patients have mourned the years of lost opportunities to change their lives as they're being checked into an operating room or angioplasty suite. We must not wait for the axe to fall. Be proactive. Change your life. Avoid coronary disease—it can be done!

Table 1 details natural practices that will keep all of our hearts healthy. Keep them in mind as you make your journey through this work, and by the time you have completed it, you will not only have learned a great deal about your heart in health and disease, but will also be well on your way to preventing heart disease in yourself and those you love. Join me now on a thrilling journey to discover how our hearts work, and how we can fix them—using both natural means and traditional medicine—when they ail.

TABLE 1
Natural Ways to Keep Our Hearts Healthy

Diet	• Low in saturated fats • High in fiber • High in fruits and vegetables • Low in trans-fatty acids • Consume cold water fish frequently (2–3 times a week): salmon, mackerel, sardines • Consume animal fats infrequently • Consume nuts frequently • Use olive oil as your oil of choice in cooking
Exercise	• 30–40 minutes of aerobic exercise 3–5 times a week • Flexibility training • Resistance training Be *certain* to check with your doctor before beginning *any* new exercise program.
Stress Reduction	• Meditation • Yoga • T'ai Chi • Freeze frame (Practice! Practice! Practice!)
Daily Multivitamins/ Multiminerals/ Supplements	• Vitamin C (1,000–2,000 mg) • Beta-carotene (5,000 IU) • L-carnitine (300 mg) • Coenzyme Q-10 (30 mg) • Natural Vitamin E (600 IU) • Alpha lipoic acid (30 mg) • Grape seed extract (40 mg) • Vitamin B_2 (20 mg) • Vitamin B_6 (50 mg) • Vitamin B_{12} (400 mcg) • Thiamin (50 mg) • Folate (1,000 mcg) • Magnesium (300 mg) • Calcium (300 mg) • Copper (2 mg)

TABLE 1 (Continued)
Natural Ways to Keep Our Hearts Healthy

Daily Multivitamins/ Multiminerals/ Supplements	• Zinc (20 mg) • Chromium (200 mcg) • Selenium (200 mcg)
Schedule regular visits with your physician	• This will maximize the likelihood of *early* detection of coronary disease, which is essential to limiting the potentially *irreversible* damage of this disorder.
Be aware of your own body and mind	• Gum disease may be a clue to underlying heart disease. • Ulcers may also be more prevalent in heart disease patients. • High stress requires immediate attention—remove as many stressors from your life as you can, and learn to employ stress reduction techniques to deal with the ones you can't eliminate.
Quit smoking! Lose weight!	• I know this advice is easier given than taken, but please believe me when I tell you that these two are *killers!*
Learn to limit anger, and nurture love and affection in your life	• Studies are now showing that anger is a physically destructive emotion, and that love can, in some cases, cure. Our hearts may not be the sole physical source of our emotions, but our emotions affect the health of our hearts—so learn to cultivate emotions that have a positive influence on your life and your heart.

CHAPTER 2

The Heart in Harmony

What gives us the drive to dissect and comprehend the workings of the heart? Is it because 42 percent of all Americans die of heart disease? Superficially, this would appear to be so, but history tells us something different. Throughout the ages, when heart disease was an anomaly rather than the norm, we have been aware of the heart's mysterious connection to our feelings. Assumed to be the seat of our emotions, the heart has been a frequent image in the poetry and literature of the past two or three millennia.

What gives the heart this special place among our organs? The heart itself does. It is clearly distinct from all other internal organs, and it tells us so. The heart is one of only two internal organs that we actually feel as it works; the other is the gut. (Interestingly, the gut also has a connection with our emotions: "I feel it in my gut.") Under rare circumstances, we can feel our hearts beating when we are calm—for instance, people lying in bed often hear their own hearts at work. More commonly, we sense our hearts at emotionally heightened moments. Recall your first kiss, how your heart seemed to swell in your chest until it was "ready to burst" with elation and clarity. The heart is truly a remarkable organ.

Not all of what it feels is great, however. Close your eyes (after you have finished reading the rest of this sentence) and recall any moment of terror, when you feared for yourself or for someone you love. Your heart will recall the pain of possible loss or perhaps the explosive racing that often precedes a "fight or flight." Whatever the feeling, the point is that you feel it, and you feel it in your heart.

Recently, researchers in the new field of psychoneuroimmunology—the study of "the mind-body connection"—have found the heart to possess qualities of intelligence, not emotion. At first glance this may appear impossible, in light of the emotional forces we imagine to be woven so deeply within the fibers of the heart. But before we prematurely draw erroneous conclusions, let us examine this more closely.

These scientists claim that, through a technique called "freeze frame," you can access the heart's intelligence. By doing so, you can resolve conflicts with greater clarity, for one. Simply stated, the "freeze frame" process works as follows: In the moment of an unproductive emotional experience (for instance, frustration and fury when not being understood), focus attention on your heart, recall a wonderful, loving experience, and then listen to your heart's response.

The process may sound strange, but I have practiced the technique and it works. When taxed by a decision I must make or conflict I must resolve, I first listen to my heart. I close my eyes and recall, for instance, the births of my children. I imagine their emergence from my wife's womb—their soft, beautiful, pink, crying bodies, little beings brimming with life and potential. The sense of gentleness and love that the image returns to me, and the inner peace that I achieve as a result, makes my work that much easier to accomplish. When relieved of the oppressive, constricting chains of confusing emotions, you too can become free to find your way. "Freeze frame" is a technique well worth trying.

Is there a contradiction here? On the one hand, millennia of great writers and thinkers tell us that the heart houses our emotions. On the other hand, recent evidence points to the heart's intellectual qualities. Which is it? The answer—both. This is what makes the heart so great. I believe that, by housing both intellect and emotion, our hearts are, in fact, organs of intuition. After all, intuition is a higher sense that embodies the union of intellect and emotion. Where emotion or intellect alone often fails, intuition comes to the fore. Intuition—the sixth sense that will most certainly evolve further during the next millennium—resides (at least partially) in that compact, dynamic powerhouse we call our heart.

Although it can be scientifically difficult to explain, "intuitive medicine" also exists. I can attest to this myself, at least in terms of my patient Mrs. June Silverstein. I was called in to the hospital to see

Mrs. Silverstein, who, as many times before, was admitted with unstable angina, an extremely serious condition. Mrs. Silverstein is a pleasant, intellectually active 88-year-old with coronary disease and gallstones. She is frequently admitted to the hospital for chest pain, and has occasionally had heart rhythm disturbances. On this admission, I went to see her as usual. In the midst of our conversation, which had dealt solely with the issue of her chest discomfort, I developed a sense of fear and understanding somewhere in the region of my heart. I suddenly understood that Mrs. Silverstein was suffering from cancer—a cancer involving her liver. At that moment, I did not know what to say to her. Instead, I rapidly concluded our conversation and ran to see her chart. Furiously flipping the pages, I found that, in fact, she had just been diagnosed with a cancer involving the ducts of her liver.

After digesting this news, I returned to her room to conclude my examination. I must say that I was astonished and perplexed by my awareness of her illness. I am not quite sure how it occurred, but I know that it happened. At no time in our conversation had she mentioned the cancer, and I'd not yet seen it described in her chart. In fact, when I was called to see her, I was simply told that she had recurrent chest pain just as she'd had on numerous previous occasions. Nevertheless, when I saw her, I knew intuitively that the cancer was present—and I "felt" that knowledge in my heart.

The heart—chambers of intellect, emotions, and intuition—is also the organ of life. Every specialist in medicine believes "his" organ to be the most important, and in this regard, cardiologists are no different. The only difference between the cardiologists' viewpoint and that of all other specialists, however, is that the heart doctors are right!

The heart is our central organ. It is the fountain of life. In addition to its spiritual, emotional, and intellectual qualities, it possesses profound physical, electrical, and mechanical properties. These latter, seemingly baser attributes allow all of us to live and breathe. Let's now examine the heart as a physical structure—a beautifully engineered, electrically driven pump.

Figure 1 helped me understand cardiac function and anatomy when I was a student at Columbia Medical School. I hope it does the same for you.

You can see that, when uncoiled, the heart is simply a tube with four valves that direct "clean" blood one way and "dirty" blood an-

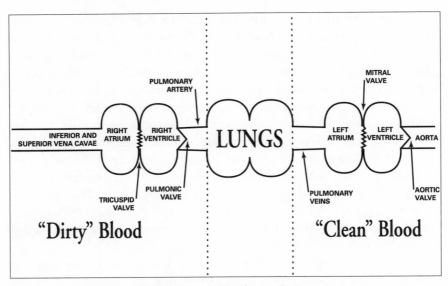

The Heart and Circulatory System

other. Blood that has been drained of nutrients and oxygen returns to the right atrium via the veins. It then passes through the right ventricle, where it is forcefully propelled toward the lungs. In the lungs, the blood is "rejuvenated" and "cleansed." It is then sent back to the left side of the heart, where it can be directed to the brain and body to deliver nourishment. In this light, the heart is really a central way station—a place where "clean" and "dirty" blood are separated and routed to their appropriate destinations.

The body possesses over 100 trillion cells which depend upon the heart's healthy function for survival. Beating 30,000 times each day, day after day, month after month, year after year, the heart has an awesome responsibility. Although it possesses many complexities, structurally it is beautifully simple, and its simplicity is what makes it such a dependable and endurable organ.

Let's now dissect the heart a little more precisely. Considering its power and immense value, the heart is a small organ. It weighs less than a pound in an average-sized man. Surrounding it is a thin, smooth, two-layered sac called the "pericardium." Filling the pericardium is a small body of fluid helping to coat the two layers so they may glide effortlessly over each other. This sac helps not only to protect the heart, but also to allow it to fill and empty, beat after beat, in a smooth and frictionless fashion.

Internally, the heart is divided into four chambers. There are two atria, thin-walled "upper chambers" that serve as blood depots. The right atrium collects "dirty" or unoxygenated blood from the veins (when the body and brain use oxygen, they take it from the arterial blood; the "used" or "dirty" blood is then returned to the heart via the veins). The left atrium receives "clean" or oxygenated blood from the lungs. Neither atrium is particularly muscular. They both serve mainly as receptacles for incoming blood.

During the period of "diastole"—when the heart rests between beats—the valves between the atria and ventricles remain open. This allows blood to travel unimpeded from right atrium to right ventricle, and left atrium to left ventricle. Just prior to ventricular squeezing, or "systole," the atria produce their own small squeeze to deliver a little extra blood to their respective ventricles. When the ventricles finally contract in systole, the valves between the atria and ventricles shut. Their closure precludes passage of blood backward from ventricles to atria. Thus, the course of blood through the cardiac chambers is one-way—i.e., once you are in the system, there is no turning back.

The valves that separate the atria and ventricles are called "atrioventricular valves." The right one is known as the tricuspid valve (having three leaflets), while the left is referred to as the mitral valve (possessing two leaflets and being shaped like a bishop's miter).

Ventricular systole—when the ventricles contract—represents the real power of the heart. When you feel your pulse, whether in your neck or wrist, you are sensing a reflection of ventricular squeezing (or systole). This beat sends the blood throughout your body, feeding and cleansing every cell. As with the atria, there are two ventricles in our heart. The right ventricle receives blood from the right atrium. It then ejects blood toward the lungs, through the pulmonic valve into the pulmonary artery. Since the pulmonary vascular system exists at low pressures, the right ventricle does not need to generate extreme force when it pumps. In fact, the peak pressure that the right ventricle generally generates is only around 25 mm of mercury.

Compare this to the left side of the heart: The left ventricle, receiving blood from the left atrium, ejects blood through the aortic valve, into the aorta, and then onward to the body and brain for sustenance. When the left ventricle squeezes, it generates much higher pressures, 120–140 mm of mercury. The pressure formed from the left ventricular squeeze is reflected in the upper reading of our blood pressure—that is, the systolic blood pressure we all worry about when we visit our doctors.

What we have just learned is that our hearts are exquisite pumps that deliver enriched blood into arteries, a network of major and minor thoroughfares which feed every cell in the body. The depleted blood is then returned toward the heart via a separate array of vessels called veins. Once in the heart, the blood can be reenriched and recirculated as the heart routes it to the lungs and then back to the rest of the body. All pumps, whether natural or artificial, require an energy supply and a control mechanism (or an on/off switch). The heart is no different.

Of course, the heart is made up of cells, and we know that all cells require blood in order to survive and function appropriately. Thus the heart, like the rest of the body, has its own blood supply—the coronary arteries. There are generally three coronary arteries (a very small number of people have four): the right, left anterior descending, and left circumflex. Each represents a distinct highway to a par-

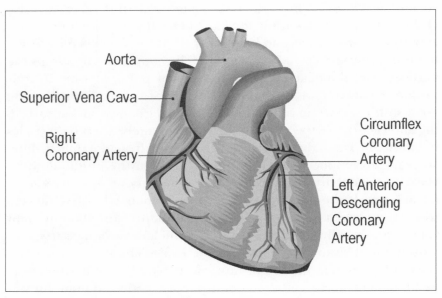

The Coronary Arteries

ticular portion of the heart. Unfortunately, there is no significant network of side roads, so if a complete blockage occurs in one of these vessels, it can result in a heart attack. Such an attack has consequences attached to it, the least of which is the death of the portion of the heart dependent upon that artery for food. I will discuss this in much greater detail in Chapter 6.

The three coronary arteries emerge from the aorta and then rest upon the surface of the heart. They send branches which arborize: dividing, subdividing, and sub-subdividing. They penetrate the heart muscle and provide blood to each of the cells that participates in making this organ the powerhouse of the body.

We know the heart is a dynamic organ, and we understand how essential it is in sustaining our lives. But what makes it tick? What times our heartbeats so precisely and perfectly throughout the years of our lives? The answer: electricity. Our hearts are fed by blood, just as our cars are fueled by gasoline—but the spark that begins each heartbeat is an electric one. The heart possesses a complex network of electrical "wires" which rapidly disseminate a single spark, resulting in the superb synchrony of every one of its beats.

Lying in the right atrium, at the level of the superior vena cava (the great vein that is the superhighway from the brain to the right atrium), is the sinoatrial node (the S-A node). This is the heart's natural pacemaker. Each of its cells is programmed to fire 60–100 times a minute. In fact, if you remove these cells from the heart and place them in a petri dish, they continue to fire every second. They are born to beat. When the S-A node fires, it sends its electric current throughout the atria. As the atria and ventricles are actually separated by fibrous (non-cellular) material, the only way for the electrical impulse to reach the ventricles is through specialized cells that function like electrical wiring. At first glance, this may appear to be an error in the great cardiac master plan. In fact, this routing of the electric current through specialized cells is actually a protective mechanism. It allows for precise and reproducible synchrony in ventricular contraction, or beats. Without synchrony, there would be chaotic and irregular squeezing of the heart, resulting in ineffectual movement of blood. The result would be disastrous.

Let's return, though, to the specialized "wiring" in the heart for a moment. The electric impulse from the S-A node has made its way through the atria to the atrioventricular node (A-V node). This node is a kind of electric filter; it creates a slight pause before allowing the impulse to pass into the HIS bundle (the "wire" that penetrates the fibrous separation of atria and ventricles). From the HIS bundle, the electric current passes to the bundle branches (left and right) prior to arborizing into a vast system of minor "wires" called Purkinje fibers, ultimately causing that explosive, perfectly coordinated delivery of electricity that causes the heart to beat.

This, then, is the anatomy of the heart. It is an elegantly designed machine or pump that routes life-sustaining blood throughout our bodies. At the same time, there is also much depth to our hearts. Housing our emotions, intellect and intuition, the heart is both simple and complex. On some levels it is precisely understood. On others, it is an enigma that will keep us wondering for eons. No matter how we look at it, it is certainly a fascinating and spectacular organ.

Heart Tests: Understanding Them Will Dissolve Your Fears

Heart tests often seem terrifying to us. How painful or dangerous will the upcoming examination be, and more anxiety-provoking yet, what will it find? Since nearly every American, at some time in his or her life, will endure one or more heart tests, it's important that we discuss them. Understanding these tests will also help us to diminish, even melt away our fears. At the same time, we should be grateful that we live in a land where health is a top priority. We are blessed with access to technologically advanced tests that are often as revealing as they are life prolonging.

Nor should it seem out of place to discuss such high-tech, invasive exams in a naturally oriented health book. Remember, my goal is to practice *integrative* cardiology. Even if a cardiovascular ailment can be treated by using alternative modalities—for instance, lowering an individual's elevated cholesterol by using niacin, garlic, and other supplements instead of a cholesterol-lowering drug—it's important to diagnose the condition properly. An undiagnosed, or improperly diagnosed, heart condition cannot be effectively managed using any system of medicine. And because untreated coronary artery disease can be fatal, we must attack it as quickly and effectively as possible, which means obtaining an accurate, timely diagnosis.

But what's it like to endure these tests? Let's follow a patient who undergoes a multitude of heart exams. Please do not infer that all patients must experience such a diversity of tests. I have invoked a bit of poetic license here at the expense of our partially fictitious patient.

My heart went out to Martha Lee, an attractive, 60-year-old

brunette, who exuded a sense of superficial confidence while re-counting what brought her to my office. Yet even before she spoke, I understood something else about her: she was afraid. And as she told her story, it became more and more obvious that, despite her exter-nal calm, Martha *knew:* she knew that today's exam would bring her awful news. Unfortunately, she was right.

Mrs. Lee came to me because of a series of new symptoms that had emerged over the past two to three months. The most troubling of her complaints was a burning in the throat that occurred after eat-ing, with extreme exertion, and during times of emotional turmoil. Her family physician had prescribed Prilosec, a medication intended to treat gastroesophageal reflux (which is essentially heartburn). When the medicine failed to eradicate her pain, Mrs. Lee sought an-other opinion without first notifying her doctor of her continued distress. I, the second opinion, had the benefit of the first doctor's failed prescription, which made my job infinitely easier.

Mrs. Lee and I spoke at great length. We talked about her father, who had died of a massive heart attack at the young age of 47. We dis-cussed her troubling cigarette addiction and her aggressive exercise program which she pursued as a talisman to ward off the spirits of her genes and tobacco use. She anguished about her two sons who, both in their thirties, were growing fat as they traded exercise for fast-paced jobs intended to bring themselves and their young fami-lies future financial security.

Mrs. Lee not only saw herself, but her two sons as well, following in her father's footsteps. We talked on. In addition to her throat dis-comfort, she had recently developed annoying palpitations—occa-sional, irregular beats of her heart which she also felt in her throat. These episodes would come without warning once or twice a week, leaving her more frightened than physically ill.

After completing her history, I took Mrs. Lee into another room to perform a physical examination, which was most revealing. She had several physical findings that pointed to the presence of signifi-cant vascular disease. I could hear high-pitched abnormal sounds (bruits) in the artery feeding the right side of her brain (the carotid artery) as well as in the artery feeding her left leg (left femoral artery). The pulses I should have been able to feel in her left foot were absent. Both of these signs—the bruits and absent pulses—in-dicated that significant plaques had already developed in her arteries, impeding the flow of blood there. Other findings of significance were a mildly elevated blood pressure of 160/90 and a faint or "soft"heart murmur, heard best over the area of her aortic valve.

After completing the history and physical examination, we performed an electrocardiogram (ECG or EKG), a test that is part of every cardiac evaluation. The EKG is an old test, dating back to 1903, when the heart's powerful electrical activity was first recorded. By appropriately positioning a series of ten electrodes on the chest, arms, and legs, we are now safely able to record the heart's electrical forces on paper.

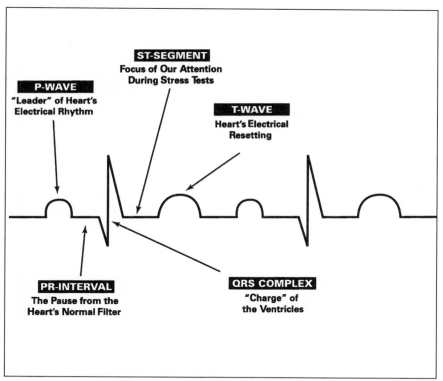

The Electrocardiogram (ECG)

There are several major waveforms that doctors evaluate. They are:

- the P-wave
- the PR interval
- the QRS complex

- the ST segment
- the T-wave

The electrical forces of the atria are represented by the P-wave—the initiator of normal cardiac cycles. The time between the end of the P-wave and the beginning of the QRS complex is termed the "PR interval." It represents the crucial pause caused by a normally functioning atrioventricular node.

The QRS complex depicts the electrical activity of the ventricles which, once stimulated, produce the major squeeze of the heart.

Occurring after the QRS complex is the "ST segment," which is the major focus of attention during exercise stress testing.

The T-wave follows the ST segment. During the T-wave, the heart is "repolarized"—its electrical charge is changed—so that it is ready to accept its next electrical impulse and, thus, its next beat. Then the electrical cycle begins all over again, as the heart continues to beat, and beat, and beat.

The EKG, a safe and painless evaluation, takes only seconds to perform and represents but a momentary glimpse of our heart's electrical power. As a result, it cannot reveal our heart's whole story, but it can provide immensely valuable information. For instance, the EKG can reveal the presence of prior heart attacks. Believe it or not, 25 percent of all heart attacks are "silent"—they have occurred in the absence of any symptoms. It is a heart-wrenching task to have to inform a "symptomless" patient that he or she is actually suffering from potentially life-threatening heart disease. These silent heart-attack victims must often go on to endure many of the exams described in this chapter. Actively evolving heart attacks, which require immediate hospitalization and dramatic therapeutic interventions, can also be diagnosed with a simple EKG, as can electrical "shorts" and occasional heart rhythm disturbances. My patient's EKG was totally normal. A normal EKG, although better than an abnormal one, does not preclude the presence of underlying heart disease.

After completing the history and physical examination, we discussed my findings and recommendations. This was the hard part for us both. If you recall, Mrs. Lee had arrived in my office superficially calm but full of fear underneath. I was now about to inform her that her fears were justified. I told her that she probably had coronary artery disease and peripheral vascular disease. I also told her that she would require a series of tests to sort out her problems and, ultimately, help me in forming an appropriate treatment strategy. Each of these tests would clarify a different piece of her medical puzzle. Again, once all the pieces were appropriately positioned, I would be more capable of rendering an intelligent and purposeful medical opinion.

Before leaving my office, I gave Mrs. Lee the first in her series of tests: an event recorder. When patients complain about palpitations, initially we want to know which are harmless (benign) and which are potentially life-threatening (malignant). Of course, the best way to do this is by actually *seeing* the heart rhythm the moment the palpitations strike. EKGs are perfect recording mechanisms here but it's obviously impractical to keep our patients hooked up until they develop symptoms. The solution: miniaturization for patient use at home.

There are two types of miniature EKG recording systems now in use: Holter monitors and event recorders. Holter monitors, the bulkier of the two, are boxes carried on shoulder straps and with chest electrodes. The Holter can continuously record the heart's rhythm for twenty-four or forty-eight hours. They are wonderful devices for patients with daily symptoms, but much less effective for patients like Martha Lee, who experienced symptoms more infrequently. As a result, I prescribed an event recorder for her.

Event recorders are smaller, lighter-weight Holters which record several minutes of our hearts' rhythms. They then erase that recording and begin a new several-minute run. The device can be worn for months, enabling us to wait for those infrequent but annoying palpitations. When a patient finally senses palpitations, he or she can trigger the device, recording the rhythm prior to and following the moment of triggering. The event is stored and then transmitted via telephone, so that it can be placed on paper and faxed to the doctor's office for immediate interpretation and attention.

During times of physical activity (e.g., tennis, golf, or sexual intercourse) when some patients have their only palpitations, I encourage them to wear both types of recording monitors. This was not necessary in Mrs. Lee's case; she wore the event recorder for only one week and experienced two episodes of palpitations. Fortunately, they were both "benign" rhythm disturbances, so she had one less worry on her mind.

Mrs. Lee's next stop was the noninvasive laboratory to undergo three separate studies. Noninvasive labs or "imaging centers" are located either within hospitals or in special offices in other buildings elsewhere. They house equipment to evaluate the inner workings of our bodies without exposing us to the risks inherent in surgery, for example. MRI, CAT scans, and ultrasound equipment, the workhorses of these centers, are harmless, painless, and often very informative.

Mrs. Lee's day of noninvasive testing began with an echocardiogram (ECHO), a very "fancy" ultrasound. All ultrasounds work on the same basic principle. When sound waves are sent to different structures, they bounce back with varying intensities, depending on the type of and distance to the structure that they strike. The pattern of their return to the recording device results in an image of either a physical structure or of blood flow.

I ordered an echocardiogram for Mrs. Lee to clarify several aspects of her condition. First, if you recall, she had a "soft murmur"—an abnormal sound of blood flow across a heart valve. Echocardiograms are the best test for evaluating heart valve abnormalities. With an enhanced computer program (called color flow Doppler), we can actually see a colorful representation of blood as it flows across our heart valves. We can also visualize the actual structure of our valves, enabling us to discern when valves are calcified, torn, infected, or narrowed. With modern echocardiography, cardiologists are able to discover minute details of the structure and function of valves.

For Mrs. Lee, the ECHO demonstrated mild calcification of an otherwise normal aortic valve. This valvular thickening is a common and usually harmless condition called "aortic sclerosis." It does not require surgery or pharmacologic agents. She clearly did not have a significant leak or narrowing of any of her four valves.

If the ECHO had been less conclusive with regard to her valves, Mrs. Lee might have been a candidate for a transesophageal echocardiogram (TEE). With the TEE, instead of placing the Doppler probe on the chest wall, it is positioned at the tip of a long tube, which is then swallowed. With the probe resting within the esophagus (the pipe connecting the mouth to the stomach), we can view the heart from *behind*. The TEE is the only cardiac exam that I have never attempted to perform. I have witnessed this examination, however, and as disturbing as it might sound, patients do tolerate it quite well. Actually, patients are sedated with intravenous medications prior to the procedure, and the fifteen- or twenty-minute exam usually passes without a hitch. If your doctor recommends this test, it may be extraordinarily beneficial for your health.

You might remember that when I evaluated Mrs. Lee in my office, I performed an EKG, which did not reveal any evidence of a previous heart attack. The ECHO is a far better test for assessing overall heart muscle function. It also will often clearly depict not only the presence of a prior heart attack, but also the location and extent of the damage. Once again Mrs. Lee was fortunate. She had no evidence of heart damage—her heart muscle was beating perfectly normally.

Other revelations were brought to light by my patient's ECHO. All of her chambers—left and right atria, left and right ventricles—were of normal size. Her heart muscle was not excessively thickened, a problem common to patients with long-standing high blood pressure (hypertension). There was no evidence of a tumor (tumors are rare but certainly potentially important discoveries). Additionally, no clots were visible within her heart. In patients with weak heart muscles, or abnormal rhythms like atrial fibrillation (see Chapter 8), clots are sometimes noted in the left ventricle or left atrium. When identified, clots often lead to a change in medication, including the addition of Coumadin, a powerful blood thinner.

During echocardiography another structure we evaluate is the pericardium—the thin, slippery, double-layered lining of the heart. When patients experience a painful inflammation of the pericardium, with the ECHO we can often visualize the excess fluid inside it. We can occasionally witness thickening or even calcification of this structure as well. Once again, my patient had no evidence of a pericardial problem. All in all, her ECHO was nearly normal, and she walked away from this test with a smile on her face.

In general, we have learned that echocardiograms have extremely broad applicability. In fact, they probably possess the widest usefulness of all cardiac tests. We can assess heart valve and muscle function, pericardial abnormalities, tumors, and clots with this one quick, safe, and painless examination.

Mrs. Lee's next study was a carotid ultrasound, specifically to determine whether or not significant plaque resided within her brain-nourishing carotid arteries. As you know, my physical examination had revealed a high-pitched noise (bruit) over her right carotid artery. This sound had raised the possibility of a silent, but potentially brain-threatening, blockage in her blood vessel. The carotid ultrasound, like the cardiac ECHO, uses sound waves to assess blood flow in the carotid arteries. Abnormal flow patterns can reveal the severity and location of blockages.

Mrs. Lee's test uncovered a moderate (50–70%) blockage (stenosis) in her right carotid artery. Since asymptomatic patients with moderate blockages in a single carotid artery are usually treated conservatively, Mrs. Lee was once again fortunate. Aspirin and cautious observation were all that she required. To decrease the likelihood of a future problem, however, she would have to make certain lifestyle changes (to be described in later chapters). Fortunately, at least for now, Mrs. Lee was spared the trauma of having to undergo surgery, an approach usually reserved for more severe blockages (stenoses) or for patients experiencing symptoms such as difficulty with speech or weakness on one side of the body.

Our patient's final test, during what was certainly a long, tiring, but enlightening day, was an assessment of the arteries feeding her legs. Once again, you will recall from Mrs. Lee's physical examination that I found a bruit (an abnormal sound) over her left femoral artery (the artery in the groin feeding the left leg). Also, I failed to detect blood pulses in her left foot. As a result, I needed to obtain a more objective analysis of the vessels supplying nourishment to her left leg, and suggested she have a test to calculate "ankle-branchial indices." By inflating cuffs at different sites along the legs, we can determine variations in pressures from the thigh all the way down to the toes. Some variations allow us to locate arterial blockages in different portions of the leg.

Based on the results of her study, I felt Mrs. Lee had a single, but significant, blockage high in her leg at the level of her left femoral artery (in the groin). Since she was asymptomatic (no leg pain with walking), and as her left foot did not demonstrate any imminent danger, surgery and angioplasty were unnecessary. Once again, I was able to treat Mrs. Lee conservatively.

The stress test was our next stop on Martha's cardiovascular circuit. Of all the "non-invasive" cardiac tests, stress tests clearly worry more patients than any other examination. There are several possible reasons why. Perhaps it's the fact that patients need to take an active role in the exam. Will I be able to walk or run enough? Will my doctor stop the treadmill if I can't go on? Will I make a fool of myself by not knowing *how* to walk on the treadmill? Could it also simply be the "unknown" that plays upon patients here? Will something be uncovered during the exam that will require additional (and more invasive) procedures? Whatever the specific reasons are that patients worry over, stress tests can be frightening experiences. So, let's try to remove some of the unnecessary concerns that plague patients by separating fact from fiction.

First, a stress test is true to its name: an examination that "stresses" the cardiovascular system. During the Master's two-step exam, the oldest stress test now rarely used, the patient walks up and down a simple step stool while having his or her EKG, blood pressure, and heart rate monitored. Although the two-step was effective, it clearly had its orthopedic limitations—walking up and down rapidly on a step stool can be very difficult for many patients.

The next rung on the evolutionary ladder of stress tests involved use of a treadmill, certainly more accessible for the vast majority of patients. Although numerous treadmill protocols have been devised, the Bruce protocol (named after Dr. Bruce, who developed it) is the most common.

The Bruce protocol uses a series of three-minute stages. The exam begins with the belt at a grade of ten degrees and a speed of 1.7 MPH. After three minutes, it jumps to 12 degrees and 2.5 MPH. Three minutes later, it is raised to 14 degrees and 3.4 MPH. Again, three minutes later (if you're still on the belt), it goes to 16 degrees and 4.2 MPH. For those extraordinarily rare ones among us who can last over 12 minutes, stage 5 is 5 MPH at 18 degrees. This stage, needless to say, is extremely difficult to perform. Rarely do patients reach this level. In fact, if you make it ten minutes or longer on the Bruce protocol, prognostically, you have a very optimistic future.

So what does a cardiologist look for as he or she observes you on the treadmill? As you walk (and sometimes run), your heart rate and blood pressure are continuously being monitored. Your EKG is also being constantly observed. The doctor carefully assesses a complete (12-lead) EKG minute by minute, especially attentive to the ST segments (the straight lines that follow QRS complexes). When these segments drop too low below the baseline, coronary artery disease can be inferred.

Inferred is the operative word here. This is *not* a diagnostic test. In other words, the stress test can be wrong. In fact, in many circumstances, this test is wrong, as much as 30–40 percent of the time. Patients with normal tests can have coronary disease, and those with abnormal tests may be free of disease. In effect, the stress test operates as a screening exam. If the EKG is normal, we are *generally* happy. If it is abnormal, we are *often* uncertain and, therefore, proceed to other more definitive exams. Nonetheless, the EKG stress test does serve a useful, even dual function as a screening exam and a measure of patient conditioning.

Nuclear stress tests, which include the use of radioactive substances, are much more accurate examinations. During these tests, very tiny amounts of radio-labeled substances (isotopes) are injected into a vein at the peak of exercise. The liquid then circulates to the heart, where it is transiently (and harmlessly) incorporated into the heart muscle. Immediately following the exercise, the patient is laid upon a table under a "gamma camera." This camera has the unique property of being able to record a picture of the heart as it absorbs emissions from the radioactive material. The imaging portion of the test lasts about twelve to twenty minutes. The pictures obtained from this segment of the study are appropriately dubbed "stress images." For completeness, "rest images" must also be taken. These are pictures taken at rest, either prior to or following the exercise portion of the exam, when the heart is calm, relaxed, and working at a much more leisurely pace.

As in the case with stress images, during the rest examination radioactive material must again be injected to reveal how the heart accepts it. The premise is as follows: Blood reaches the heart through coronary arteries. Coronary arteries feed specific segments of the heart. The radioactive material is briefly incorporated into the heart muscle only when it can reach it by passing through the coronary arteries. During exercise, the heart beats faster and harder, requiring substantially more nourishment (in the form of blood flow) to sustain itself. When an artery is partially plugged with plaque, it may provide adequate blood flow at rest. With exercise, however, the stiffened and diseased artery may not be as capable.

As a result, a discrepancy arises between the contrasting images in a nuclear stress test. With the patient at rest, the images appear normal as the heart receives ample blood flow and the nuclear agent lodges itself evenly throughout the heart muscle. With the patient undergoing the stress of exercise, however, the images appear abnormal—with abnormality defined as a paucity of the radioactive isotope visible in the particular segment of the heart being fed by a partially blocked artery.

This finding is called "ischemia"; it represents a lack of blood flow to a portion of the heart. It can be contrasted with a heart attack (myocardial infarct), which represents a dead area of the heart. When an infarct exists, the nuclear agent can never be incorporated within that area of heart muscle, neither during exercise nor at rest.

Nuclear stress tests have significantly improved the accuracy of the stress examination. They are correct 80–90 percent of the time. In other words, they are wrong only 10–20 percent of the time. It must be remembered, though, that these tests are also *inferential* exams. We are often confident of our diagnoses, but we are definitely not certain of them.

Before briefly discussing a "non-exercise" type of stress test, I must allay any fears you might have regarding the safety of the actual stress portion of this test. It is extremely safe. In fact, the risk of dying during a stress test is less than 1 in 10,000. So please, try not to be riddled with fear as you step on the treadmill for your stress test.

For those patients who are unable to walk adequately (or for those patients with an EKG abnormality termed left bundle branch block—see Chapter 8), we often perform resting stress tests. During these exams, we attempt to simulate exercise by administering intravenous medications like Adenosine or Dobutamine.

Adenosine is a drug which dilates normal coronary arteries but does not do the same for abnormal (or plaque-filled) vessels. When infused, it creates a different blood flow to cardiac segments fed by normal and abnormal vessels. Normal vessels receive better flow. Once again, through the use of radioactive helpers, we can visualize this blood-flow variation and often diagnose coronary artery disease.

Dobutamine is a drug that increases the heart rate and strength of muscle squeezing, also simulating exercise. This drug is often infused intravenously during "sedentary" stress tests done with echocardiography rather than nuclear imaging. If you recall from our discussion of ECHOs, these tests can accurately assess heart muscle function. Segments of the heart walls squeeze poorly when deprived of blood flow. During times of rest, a segment fed by a partially plugged artery may function perfectly well. With exercise, however, localized inadequate blood flow may leave this area of the heart hungry, resulting in a diminished capacity to squeeze. This change in heart muscle function can often be discerned during a stress ECHO, whether the stress is pharmacologic (i.e., caused by Dobutamine) or caused by exercise.

At this point, I must also touch upon two tests which screen for the presence of coronary artery disease and which I am often questioned about: the PET scan and the ultrafast CT scan. The PET (which stands for "positron emission tomography") scan is an extremely costly way to assess the heart's metabolism. In detecting reduced blood flow (ischemia), it has a minimally improved accuracy over the more typical nuclear tests just described, perhaps only by 10 percent. Thus, the PET scan is more of an experimental rather than clinical tool.

The ultrafast (or electron beam) CT has also been touted as a major breakthrough in coronary artery disease detection. Some have suggested it will supplant angiography. Unfortunately, it won't. The test searches for abnormal calcium deposits within the coronary arteries. Although these deposits indicate the presence of coronary artery disease, the extent of disease and the calcium deposits' prognostic implications still remain unknown. Such uncertainty calls for more studies of this technique. In this respect, the American Heart Association has not yet advocated its use as a screening tool.

But let's now return to our patient, Martha Lee, to find out what transpired during her nuclear stress test.

Mrs. Lee underwent a stress test with Cardiolite, a radioactive material. During this exam, she developed her typical throat-burning, and her EKG showed ST segment changes that were quite suggestive of reduced blood flow (ischemia). When she finished exercising, I informed her that I was very concerned about her results, but in order to be more certain of her diagnosis, we would have to wait for the results of her nuclear scan.

The pictures revealed what I had expected. Mrs. Lee had a large territory of ischemia in the front (anterior) wall of the heart. She appeared to be suffering from a tightly blocked left anterior descending artery. The good news was that her heart muscle was normal. Again there was no evidence of an earlier heart attack. Given the large and important area of her heart in jeopardy, we needed a more definitive sense of what her coronary artery anatomy looked like. Therefore I suggested that she undergo one final (and invasive) examination: a cardiac catheterization, or "angiogram."

Although I described the cardiac catheterization or coronary angiogram in Chapter 2, when Mr. Goldberg underwent his procedure, here I will briefly depict a more personal angiogram—my own.

Several years ago, I began to develop a deeply troubling symptom, exertional chest pressure which radiated to my throat and jaw. This occurred during a period when I was trying to "get back in shape." Every time I jogged, the same symptom would appear, ultimately sending me into an extreme panic. My grandfather had developed coronary artery disease at a very young age, and sharing many of his characteristics, I imagined that soon I, too, would acquire the legacy of heart disease. Therefore, I underwent many of the examinations about which you just read. I had an EKG and chest X-ray, both of which were normal. My ECHO was also normal. I then endured a non-nuclear stress test (performed by my cardiologist father-in-law). This, unfortunately, was abnormal (you can imagine how my poor father-in-law felt). To improve the accuracy of the stress exam, I had a nuclear (thallium, not Valium) stress test. Unfortunately, this test was equivocal. As an invasive cardiologist, I had but one option. If I were ever to regain my sanity and dismiss the notion that I had undiagnosed coronary artery disease, I needed to have a cardiac cathetherization (i.e., an angiogram).

Quickly, I contacted my colleague and friend, Dr. Michael Collins. After I described my symptoms and stress tests, he concurred with my assessment, and we set the date for my impending angiogram. The night before the test was sleepless. I lay awake feeling my own femoral pulse, and imagining what it would feel like to have my groin area numbed and catheters threaded into my arteries. Of course, I imagined myself experiencing every possible complication—excessive bleeding, a stroke or heart attack, and even (rare as it is) dying. I also reflected positively on the fact that this was to be a *diagnostic* test (i.e., definitive), not *inferential* (speculative) as my stress tests had been. I knew that when I returned home later that day, it would be with a sense of relief. I would know where I stood—if I had coronary artery disease or if this had just been one large, terrifying, but harmless moment in my life.

I recall my angiogram vividly. After arriving at the hospital early in the morning to have blood tests, I was taken into the catheterization laboratory, prepped and sedated. Dr. Collins then performed his task. The angiogram revealed a beautifully pristine coronary anatomy. Although I was half asleep, my scientific side was still awake, and it happily saw that my arteries were normal. After lying still for six hours—to help my body form a plug that would seal my artery closed—I went home.

I was tired but so elated. I was one of the lucky ones. With a normal angiogram, I had a clean bill of health, enabling me to resume exercise with impunity. By the way, I later discovered that my chest pain probably had resulted from mild exertional asthma—quite a workup to arrive at that realization, eh? Nevertheless, I learned much from my cardiovascular exams. I not only learned what had been causing my pain, but also discovered what it feels like to endure many heart procedures. I experienced firsthand the emotional angst which plagues so many of our patients. The experience allayed my own personal fears and enabled me to become a more compassionate and empathetic physician.

Mrs. Lee underwent her angiogram but was, sadly, not quite so fortunate as I had been. Mrs. Lee had one very tightly blocked artery. Her LAD (the vessel feeding the front wall of the heart) had a 90 percent lesion at its origin. This type of blockage can be deadly. In fact, it is often referred to as the "widow-maker" (or "widower-maker," in Mrs. Lee's case). Although this is harsh terminology, it is unfortunately accurate. Complete occlusions of this vessel often result in a massive heart attack or sudden cardiac death.

The good news was that her other arteries were fine and her heart muscle was definitely normal. The other good news was that Mrs. Lee's blockage appeared to be very approachable, and that she would be able to avoid the invasion of surgery by enduring the much less traumatic treatment of a percutaneous (through the skin in the groin) procedure. Yes, she could be treated effectively with an angioplasty and stent, which I will explore, along with other like procedures in Chapters 4 and 5.

Please keep in mind, though, that I vigorously encouraged Mrs. Lee, like all my patients, to go well beyond the approaches to her ailments just mentioned. Stress reduction techniques such as meditation, freeze frame, and yoga; resistance and aerobic exercise; and intensive nutritional modification with supplementary herbs and vitamins would be very useful to her. Remember, it is the prevention of cardiac disease—both primary (before it strikes) and secondary (after an initial event)—that is the ultimate goal of my practice. Remember, too, as you read the next chapters, that whenever possible in the management of cardiovascular disease, I attempt to incorporate the valuable remedies of a naturalist's medicine chest. The final chapters of this book will detail how you can bring these wonderful elements of health and healing into your own life.

CHAPTER 4

Heart Breakers: The Many Causes of Coronary Disease

Coronary artery disease does indeed carry grim statistics: A million-and-a-half heart attacks ("myocardial infarctions") occur annually in the United States. Almost half of them occur in people under the age of 65—often at the peak of a person's working and child-rearing years. Approximately 1 million Americans die annually from coronary artery disease, making this the number one killer in the United States, destroying cumulatively 42 percent of all Americans. The economic loss from coronary artery disease is enormous, drawing $50–$150 billion a year from our economy. What causes this beast to penetrate our lives so fiercely—ripping parents from their children, children from parents, husbands from wives, wives from husbands, friends from friends, and so on? What can we do to stop its onslaught so that we may live longer, more productive, and fulfilled lives? In the following pages I will address these and other questions.

Understanding coronary artery disease, however, does require some familiarity with the anatomy and physiology of normal coronary arteries. You will recall from Chapter 2 that there are three large arteries lying on the heart (the epicardial coronary arteries). Each one arborizes, creating networks of finer and finer arteries, arterioles, and ultimately capillaries—the smallest blood vessels.

Each artery, regardless of its size, possesses three layers. The inner layer, or intima, is lined by a single sheath of endothelial cells. These cells are in direct contact with the blood that courses through our arteries, carrying nutrients, oxygen, and a variety of cells and hormonal substances. The middle layer, or media, comprises multiple layers of smooth muscle cells and fibrous connective tissue. The outer layer, or adventitia, is made up not only of cells but also of an extensive vascular and neural (nerves) network enmeshed within dense, strong, fibrous tissue. Thus, we see that even a single artery is extraordinarily complex.

With regard to coronary artery disease, the endothelial cells, though but a single layer, carry the most weight. These cells are immensely complex, containing receptor sites for numerous substances such as LDL cholesterol, growth factors, and various pharmacologic agents. Endothelial cells also produce the most powerful dilator (expander) of blood vessels, a substance called "endothelial-derived relaxing factor" or EDRF. Recently, EDRF has been discovered to be nitric oxide, the same type of molecule that gives Viagra its kick.

This, then, is a simplified image of our arteries as they exist in health. How do they appear when ill, and what is it that makes them sick?

There are currently two theories on the cause (etiology) of coronary artery disease. The first, and more widely accepted theory—the "response to injury hypothesis"—implicates numerous factors impacting our arteries and resulting in injury. Such injuries can then initiate a series of responses, which ultimately produce severe blockages to blood flow. The second, less widely accepted theory—the "monoclonal hypothesis"—considers coronary artery disease to be closer to a cancer-like ("neoplastic") process.

Personally, I lean toward the response to injury hypothesis. It makes perfect sense, and it allows for the existence of a variety of well-established causative factors. This agrees with our current body of scientific knowledge, which has demonstrated numerous potent risk factors for coronary artery disease (soon to be discussed in great detail). As a result of any of a vast number of injuries, the same three biological processes unfold: (1) there is a migration of smooth muscle cells into the intima—a place that is normally simply a peaceful single layer of endothelial cells; (2) the connective tissue (the fibrous tissue component of the intima) increases substantially; and (3) lipids (fats) accumulate within the smooth muscle cells that have moved from the media to the intima. Lipids also accumulate within macrophages, the white blood cells that have entered the intima from the bloodstream.

All lesions (or plaques) contain varying amounts of these three elements—fats (lipids), smooth muscle cells, and fibrous tissue—but a typical plaque passes through a typical metamorphosis. The infant plaque is called the "fatty streak," and in fact, this lesion can be found in "normal" children. It is an intima that's been invaded by lipid-laden macrophages and smooth muscle cells. As time goes on, more fibrous tissue is deposited within the plaque, and thus, the lesion becomes the "fibrous plaque." This more mature blockage has been observed in autopsy studies of otherwise "healthy" young adults. As we (and our plaques) age, they can become "complex" lesions, containing calcium or even blood clots. These more complex plaques can lead to heart attacks.

Risk Factors for Coronary Artery Disease

When discussing cardiac risk factors, we must draw a distinction between modifiable and nonmodifiable risks. The term "modifiable risks" implies that we can do something about them. It is within our control to limit these risk factors and, thus, decrease our likelihood of developing coronary disease. Obviously, modifiable risk factors are the ones we must aggressively attack when trying to prevent and cure coronary disease.

"Nonmodifiable risks" are those about which we can do nothing. They include genetic predisposition, age, and gender. We do not have the ability to choose our own parents; thus, there is nothing we can do about limiting our genetic predisposition to coronary disease. (It is interesting to note the power of genes—the younger the age when developing coronary artery disease, the greater the likelihood that one's children will also suffer from the disease.)

Additionally, to my knowledge, no one has yet been successful at slowing the aging process. We all get older, and as we age, our risk for coronary disease increases. In fact, most myocardial infarctions occur in patients over the age of 65. With regard to gender, men have a higher incidence of coronary disease until women enter menopause. Shortly thereafter, women's risk for developing coronary disease increases, approaching that of men. The Framingham Heart Study, which started in the 1950s, and has followed 5,209 men and women, ages 35–94, for nearly 40 years, remains ongoing today.

It's demonstrated that men generally develop coronary artery disease ten years earlier than women. Unfortunately, after menopause, women catch up. Although modern medicine has advanced greatly, it still can do nothing to diminish these three risk factors.

Of the modifiable risk factors, we distinguish between major and minor ones. Those which have been shown to have the greatest impact on coronary disease are dubbed major, while those of lesser consequence, minor. The major risk factors are generally considered to be: high cholesterol, high blood pressure, diabetes mellitus, smoking, and a family history of coronary artery disease (a genetic and, therefore, nonmodifiable risk factor). Recently obesity was upgraded and added to this list.

The minor risk factors include: an elevated homocysteine level, elevated LPa (a type of especially "sticky" LDL) level, Type A behavior pattern, physical inactivity, a low level of circulating antioxidants, and certain hemostatic factors such as elevated fibrinogen levels. Let's now look at modifiable risk factors, starting first with high cholesterol, or hypercholesterolemia.

Hypercholesterolemia

Lipids—fats—have received very bad press during the last several decades. Some of this bad press is well deserved, since some fats can contribute to many devastating diseases. This is not the whole story, however; lipids are *essential* components of every cell in our body. Fats are necessary constituents of cell membranes, maintaining cell integrity while allowing them to communicate with the outside world. Our brains, for instance, contain a surprising amount of fat, which they require to function correctly. The point is, we all need fat; we just need to make sure we consume the right fats in the right amounts.

Fat and water don't mix—we witness this while making salad dressing. In order to have a more homogeneous mixture to apply to our salads, we need to shake the dressing vigorously. It's no different in our bodies. Blood is a water-based (or "aqueous") solution. For lipids to travel in the blood from one part of the body to another, they must be transported in structures called lipoproteins. This makes them water soluble, so they can interact with the water-based solution, that is, our blood.

TABLE 2
Risk Factors for Coronary Artery Disease

Nonmodifiable Risk Factors

Genetic predisposition	Coronary artery disease often runs in families, but just because your parents or grandparents had heart disease, that doesn't mean that you will. The younger a person develops coronary artery disease, however, the greater the likelihood that his or her children will also have heart disease.
Age	The percentage of people with coronary artery disease increases with age, and most heart attacks occur in people over the age of 65.
Gender	Men have a higher incidence of coronary artery disease than women and they generally develop it about 10 years earlier. After women enter menopause, however, their risk of heart disease approaches that of men.

Modifiable Risk Factors

Major

Elevated cholesterol	An increased level of LDL (low density lipoprotein) cholesterol is associated with developing coronary artery disease. Diet, exercise, appropriate supplementation (including gugulipid, garlic, soluble fiber, L-carnitine, and pantethine), and/or cholesterol-lowering drugs can be used to improve cholesterol levels.
High blood pressure	Every 7.5 millimeter increase in blood pressure (the diastolic blood pressure) increases the risk of heart disease by 29%. High blood pressure also increases the risk of stroke. Exercise, stress reduction techniques (such as meditation), diet, and/or medication can be used to control blood pressure. Supplements such as magnesium and coenzyme Q-10, as well as herbs such as hawthorn, coleus forskohii, and khella, can be used to help control high blood pressure.
Diabetes	Vascular disease, including heart disease, kills nearly 80% of American diabetic patients. This risk can be decreased by tightly controlling blood sugar levels through diet, appropriate supplementation (including soluble fiber, chromium, and bitter melon), exercise, and medication when required.

TABLE 2 (Continued)
Risk Factors for Coronary Artery Disease

Smoking	Research has demonstrated a marked increase in heart attack deaths in smokers: Deaths increase by 18% in men and 31% in women for every ten cigarettes smoked each day. Even using smokeless tobacco increases the risk of death from heart disease.
Obesity	Both obesity and "yo-yo" dieting have been shown to contribute to the development of cardiovascular disease. Approximately 60 million adult Americans are currently classified as obese. Weight can usually be modified by using diet and exercise. Supplements such as fiber, chromium, and coenzyme Q-10 are helpful to some people in losing weight.
Minor (but important)	
Physical inactivity	Physical inactivity can contribute to high blood pressure, weight gain, increased cholesterol levels, and even depression. Exercise decreases body weight and blood pressure, increases HDL cholesterol and blood sugar stability, and aids relaxation.
Low levels of antioxidants	Antioxidants, like vitamin E, appear to protect arteries against damage from LDL cholesterol. Therefore, having inadequate levels of antioxidants may contribute to the development of coronary artery disease. Antioxidants such as vitamins C and E, coenzyme Q-10, grape seed extract, and alpha lipoic acid are obtainable from both food and supplements.
High homocysteine levels	An increased level of this by-product of protein breakdown has recently been accepted as an important risk for coronary artery disease. Homocysteine levels can generally be controlled by taking adequate amounts of vitamins B_6, B_{12}, and the B vitamin folic acid, as well as by modifying your diet to consume less red meat.
Type A behavior pattern	While it's hard to evaluate emotions scientifically, we know that stress leads to elevated levels of cortisol and adrenaline, which have destructive effects on our bodies. Stress has been linked to development of angina and coronary artery disease, although studies disagree in their definitions of "Type A behavior" and the amount of its impact on heart disease. Stress reduction techniques like exercise, meditation, Eastern disciplines like yoga or T'ai Chi, and others can help limit the toll stress takes on our bodies. Supplements such as kava kava, St. John's wort, and valerian can be used to help induce relaxation.

TABLE 2 (Continued)
Risk Factors for Coronary Artery Disease

Increased levels of clotting factors	Elevated levels of blood clotting factors like Factor 7 and fibrinogen may contribute to the development of heart disease. The potential role in causing heart disease played by these blood factors (and others, like plasminogen activator) is still under investigation. The blood can be "thinned" by using medications and appropriate supplements, including the Omega-3 fatty acids DHA and EPA, as well as garlic and vitamin E.
High LPa (lipoprotein a)	This lipoprotein is thought to be a particularly "sticky" form of LDL cholesterol, and may therefore be a major contributor to the development of heart disease. At the present time, it appears that keeping LDL cholesterol measurements under control corrects the damaging potential of elevated LPa levels as well.

The major lipoproteins include very low density lipoproteins (VLDL, also called "chylomicrons"), intermediate density lipoproteins (IDL), low density lipoproteins (LDL), and high density lipoproteins (HDL). Our livers help metabolize (create *and* destroy) these lipoproteins.

HDL, the "good" cholesterol, is the lipoprotein that brings fat back to the liver to be metabolized. LDL, the "bad" cholesterol, is the lipoprotein that carries cholesterol to various parts of the body. When evaluating your cholesterol profile, it is the LDL number that concerns most physicians, as elevated LDL has been shown in numerous studies to increase the risk of developing coronary disease.

During my exploration of the world of natural medicine, I have learned a great deal from many of the "natural healers" of our time. I have also been exposed to a rather misguided viewpoint that seems to ignore a substantial amount of good medical literature. There are those within the world of natural medicine who feel that elevated cholesterol levels do not predispose people to coronary artery disease, and that lowering cholesterol does nothing to limit coronary artery disease. I emphatically disagree. Numerous studies demonstrate the importance of cholesterol lowering in the management of coronary disease. Natural supplements such as garlic, gugulipid, and the water-soluble fibers can be used to lower cholesterol in many cases, rather than cholesterol-lowering drugs. However you do it, though, elevated cholesterol levels must be lowered to protect your heart.

How We Know: The Studies

Observational studies—those in which large numbers of patients were observed over long periods of time, allowing us to infer cause and effect relationships—laid the groundwork for our understanding of elevated cholesterol in regard to coronary artery disease. The MRFIT (Multiple Risk Factor Intervention Trial), for instance, evaluated 350,000 men. It demonstrated that those men with elevated cholesterol had an increased risk of developing coronary disease. Other studies, such as the Seven Country Study and the Nihansan study, clearly demonstrated that nationality and ethnicity alone are not protective against coronary disease. In the Seven Country Study, for example, Finnish and U.S. patients were evaluated and found to have more frequent coronary disease when their intake of saturated fat and cholesterol was high. In the Nihansan study, Japanese men living in the United States increased their dietary intake of saturated fats and cholesterol compared to Japanese men living in Japan—and, as a result, demonstrated a much higher incidence of coronary disease than their counterparts in Japan.

These observational studies, though not the gold standard for scientific analyses, set the stage for future studies by demonstrating the probable relationship between dietary fat intake and the development of coronary disease. Interventional trials followed in which people with elevated cholesterol levels were put on cholesterol-lowering medication to determine whether lowering cholesterol would, in fact, decrease the likelihood of their developing coronary disease.

Two types of interventional trials have been performed. *Primary* prevention trials assess patients who do not have documented coronary disease, and attempt to determine whether lowering their cholesterol will also decrease their likelihood of developing future cardiovascular events. *Secondary* prevention trials analyze patients who have already developed coronary disease, in order to determine whether lowering their cholesterol will limit their likelihood of experiencing *recurrent* events.

Several of the primary prevention trials deserve special attention. The Lipid Research Clinic Coronary Primary Prevention Trial analyzed 3,800 men with hypercholesterolemia. These men were treated with either a high dose of a cholesterol-lowering drug, cholestyramine, or a placebo. A moderate dietary improvement was also made. Because of the high dose of the cholestyramine and its frequent gastrointestinal side effects, there was low compliance in taking the medication. During the seven-and-a-half-year follow-up, however, researchers found that for every 1% drop in cholesterol via dietary and drug intervention, there was a 2–3% drop in the frequency of coronary artery disease events. Overall, there *was* a decrease in the death rate from coronary disease. Unfortunately, however, due to the slightly increased risks of accidental and violent deaths, which were also factored in (but which had nothing to do with cholesterol-lowering drugs), the improvements we're concerned about were somewhat obscured.

Nor do we understand why accidental and violent deaths increased in this particular patient population, but two other studies demonstrated similar findings. The World Health Organization Cooperative Trial treated over 10,000 men with another cholesterol-lowering drug, clofibrate, or a placebo. At five and a half years, the researchers again noted a decrease in the death rate from cardiovascular disease. At the same time an increase in noncardiovascular deaths obscured the mortality benefit achieved via drug therapy. The Helsinki Heart Study, which enlisted 4,800 men with hypercholesterolemia, also found a significant reduction in coronary artery disease morbidity and mortality in those patients treated with a third cholesterol-lowering drug, gemfibrozil. In this study, researchers noted a statistically *insignificant* increase in death rate from accidental and violent causes. The West of Scotland Coronary Prevention Study evaluated 6,600 men with documented high cholesterol. These men were treated with 40 mg of Pravastatin versus placebo. In this trial cardiovascular mortality and morbidity *were* improved, and there was *no* increase in risk of death from accidental or violent causes.

Generally, these primary prevention trials all demonstrated that lowering cholesterol levels with medications diminishes the risk of developing coronary disease. These studies assessed large numbers of patients, and in my view represent enough scientific evidence for using cholesterol-lowering drugs, when necessary, to lower cholesterol levels and help prevent the development of coronary artery disease.

Secondary prevention trials have also demonstrated the efficacy of cholesterol lowering in limiting coronary artery disease. Let's focus now on some of the more interesting elements of those studies. The Coronary Drug Project was a large study, examining 8,300 men with prior heart attacks (myocardial infarctions). Significantly, researchers here demonstrated the effectiveness of a vitamin, nicotinic acid. Nicotinic acid, vitamin B_3, successfully decreased recurrences of myocardial infarctions and lowered long-term death rates at a fifteen-year follow-up. Yes, the addition of a simple vitamin can have a dramatic impact on our lives.

The first trial actually to observe angiographic benefits from lowering cholesterol was the National Heart, Lung, Blood Institute (NHLBI) Type 2 Coronary Intervention Study. In this trial, pre- and post-cardiac catheterizations were performed on 143 men and women. Patients were also treated with the drug cholestyramine, causing a significant reduction in the progression of coronary artery disease. The Canadian Coronary Atherosclerosis Intervention Trial (the CCAIT) was also quite revealing; it demonstrated, through angiography, not only a decrease in the progression of plaque with lovastatin (a cholesterol-lowering drug), but also in the development of *new* blockages.

TABLE 3
Vitamins and Supplements That May Help Prevent Coronary Artery Disease by Modifying Cholesterol

Vitamin/ Supplement	Daily Dosage	Action	Potential Side Effects
Vitamin B_3 (nicotinic acid or niacin)	1,000– 3,000 mg daily	Niacin causes the liver to make as much as 15–25% less LDL cholesterol. A 15-year study of individuals taking niacin to lower LDL cholesterol showed decreased recurrences of coronary heart disease and lowered death rates from heart attack. Niacin raises HDL more than any other agent and lowers Lp(a) levels.	• Liver abnormality. • A "flushing" sensation in the skin. • Worsening of gout, ulcer, glaucoma, glucose control in diabetics. • Muscle inflammation when combined with statins (drugs that also decrease LDL levels).

TABLE 3 (Continued)
Vitamins and Supplements That May Help Prevent
Coronary Artery Disease by Modifying Cholesterol

Omega-3 fatty acids DHA and EPA	3,000 mg (combined)	The fatty acids DHA and EPA lower triglycerides and increase HDL, the "good" cholesterol. They've also been observed to lower high blood pressure. These omega-3 fatty acids are found naturally in fatty fish (such as salmon and mackerel), and are available as supplements.	• The omega-3 fatty acids thin the blood, and so can interact in rare circumstances with other blood thinners (including aspirin) to cause bleeding.
Natural Vitamin E	400–800 IU	This antioxidant protects against oxidation of LDL cholesterol, thereby protecting arteries against harmful LDL cholesterol.	• Rare (if any) at these doses.
Alpha lipoic acid	30–100 mg	This antioxidant protects against oxidation of LDL cholesterol, thereby protecting arteries.	• May cause insomnia at high doses.
Vitamin C	1,000–2,000 mg	This antioxidant vitamin protects against oxidation of LDL cholesterol, thereby protecting arteries.	• Gastric upset in susceptible individuals. • Use with caution in kidney failure, kidney stones, and gout.
Grape seed extract	40–100 mg	This antioxidant protects arteries against harmful LDL cholesterol.	• Rare (if any) at these doses.
Pyridoxine (B_6)	50 mg	This vitamin lowers homocysteine levels.	• At sustained high doses (greater than 150 mg daily) can very rarely cause peripheral neuropathy.
Pantethine (B_5)	300 mg 3 times daily	This vitamin lowers LDL cholesterol.	
Choline	4–6 g	Lowers LDL cholesterol.	• GI upset.

Another fascinating study was the St. Thomas Atherosclerosis Regression Trial (or START). In this trial, researchers made two interventions: they used cholestyramine to lower cholesterol and increased essential fatty acids to 8 percent of the total caloric intake. In the group so treated, researchers noted regression of coronary artery disease and a decrease in cardiovascular events, supporting the use not only of drugs but also essential fatty acids in managing coronary disease. These health-promoting fats are too frequently absent from our diets, and so we'll talk about them more later.

As you can see, numerous studies have demonstrated important improvements in coronary anatomy through the use of cholesterol-lowering medications. You may, therefore, conclude that these "observable" arterial changes are necessary to reduce cardiovascular events like heart attacks. The Pravastatin Limitation of Atherosclerosis in the Coronary Arteries Trial (PLAC 1) disproved this belief, on the other hand, by demonstrating a decrease in cardiovascular events in the absence of any obvious changes in the coronary anatomy.

Seemingly, there is more than just coronary anatomy at work here. Even without any visible changes in the amount of coronary blockage, patients taking cholesterol-lowering medicines experienced a significant decline in the frequency of heart attacks. Although a picture is worth a thousand words, in this situation the picture—of the coronary blockages—is certainly not telling the whole story.

Finally, the Scandinavian Simvastatin Survival Study (the 4S study) evaluated 4,444 men and women with coronary artery disease. This landmark study documented an overall mortality reduction of 30 percent with the use of the drug Simvastatin, as well as a cardiovascular mortality reduction of 42 percent. There was no significant increase in noncardiac deaths in this study, and this trial clearly demonstrated that lipid-lowering drugs decrease mortality in patients with documented coronary artery disease.

There are many other trials that have looked at primary and secondary prevention of coronary disease through cholesterol-lowering agents. I have presented a small sample of some of the more important of these studies to give you a sense of the great body of evidence that convincingly establishes both the vital role of cholesterol lowering in the fight against coronary disease and the complexity at work here. In my own practice, I use a combination of lifestyle changes, drugs, herbs, and vitamins to achieve cholesterol lowering. Of course, I prefer using natural methods to improve my patients' health, but sometimes heart disease is so advanced by the time I see a patient that it is already life-threatening. When natural or nonpharamacologic therapy is inadequate to bring cholesterol down, I advocate drug therapy to limit cardiovascular disease and mortality.

Having reviewed several important cholesterol-lowering studies and now understanding the role of cholesterol in coronary artery disease, let's examine what can be done to limit its deadly effects, using both pharmacologic agents and natural approaches. Hypercholesterolemia is a perfect example of the need to integrate natural and traditional approaches in managing diseases. We will see that a combination of approaches embodies the ultimate solution to this (any many other) maladies.

Cholesterol-Lowering Medications

There is a plethora of pharmacologic agents aimed at lowering cholesterol levels. These drugs vary in their mechanisms of actions as well as in their efficacy. Some lower LDL more than triglycerides, others lower triglycerides more than LDL, and some raise HDL where others do not. They also possess varying side effects, and certainly these drugs should not be viewed as a homogeneous group. It generally takes two years or longer before any clinical benefits are noted from cholesterol lowering. Therefore, don't be disheartened if you or a loved one experiences a side effect, or even a cardiac-related health event, shortly after beginning to take a cholesterol-lowering drug.

Bile Acid Sequestrants

The bile acid sequestrants (ammonium salts) are often provided in a powdered form. Cholestyramine and cholestipol are the two most often prescribed bile acid sequestrant drugs. These agents work by interrupting the normal circulation of bile acids between the gut and the liver. They bind bile acids in the intestines, and so increase their excretion in the stool. As a result, more cholesterol is used to create new bile acids and blood cholesterol levels fall. These agents have been found to decrease LDL levels by 15–50 percent in some studies, with HDL minimally increased and triglycerides not usually affected. Some patients with preexisting hypertriglyceridemia (elevated triglyceride levels) can actually have a worsening of their triglycerides with the use of the bile acid sequestrants. Although no clear systemic toxicity has been noted with these drugs, they represent a potential threat to absorbing fat-soluble vitamins.

Nicotinic Acid (Niacin)

Nicotinic acid or niacin (vitamin B_3) is so effective at lowering cholesterol that, while it is a vitamin, it's also considered to be a cholesterol-lowering medication. Niacin lowers total cholesterol levels by decreasing the liver's synthesis and release of LDL cholesterol. In other words, it decreases the *formation* of LDL. Some studies have demonstrated a 15–25 percent reduction in LDL with vitamin B_3. The recommended dose is 1.5 to 6 g per day. A flushing sensation in which your skin can feel "on fire" is the factor that most commonly limits this dosage. You can ameliorate this unpleasant sensation by taking an aspirin thirty minutes prior to taking the niacin. Other possible side effects from niacin use include liver failure (extremely rare, but more common when using a sustained release form), activation of pre-existing peptic ulcer disease, an increase in the frequency of gout, worsening of glaucoma, and a worsening of glucose control in diabetic patients. A rare, but important, side effect is inflammation of the muscles, which occurs slightly more frequently when taking niacin in conjunction with drugs called HMG-CoA reductase inhibitors or statins (described below).

All that said, niacin is generally a safe medication and I have had very positive results using it in my own clinical practice. I should also note that niacin has two other "side benefits" lacking in most other cholesterol-lowering drugs. First, niacin can increase HDL levels by 15–35 percent. For every percentage increase in the HDL, there is a 2–3 percent *reduction* in cardiovascular risk. This is an extremely important effect of niacin. Niacin also can lower LPa levels. LPa is a very virulent form of LDL, and at high levels may predispose an individual to coronary disease. In fact, niacin is the most effective LPa-lowering agent currently available. I generally restrict the use of niacin to patients who have minimally elevated LDL levels and very low HDL levels or very high LPa levels. For your information as well, niacin is not a wonderful agent for lowering LDL; other drugs like the HMG-CoA reductase inhibitors are much better for this purpose.

HMG-CoA Reductase Inhibitors (Statins)

The statins work by inhibiting the enzyme HMG-CoA reductase. The result is a decrease in circulating (i.e., blood) LDL levels. It is interesting to note that plasminogen activator inhibitor 1 (PAI-1), a substance which causes an increase in our blood's clotting capacity, is also decreased with the use of HMG-CoA reductase inhibitors. This may be an added benefit of these drugs, but has not yet been evaluated to any large extent.

TABLE 4
Culinary Herbs That Help to Manage High Cholesterol

- Garlic
- Cayenne Pepper
- Turmeric
- Soluble fiber from plant sources such as:
  Guar gum
  Psyllium
  Pectin

When taking a fiber supplement, be sure that you drink plenty of water—at least one or two 8–12-ounce glasses daily with each fiber supplement.

Of all the drugs, statins are the best at lowering LDL, dropping levels by 20–40 percent of their initial values. They also slightly increase HDL levels to 5 percent or even 15 percent above baseline, and often decrease triglyceride levels about 10–20 percent.

These drugs are actually very well tolerated and patients are rarely forced to discontinue their use. Liver problems (hepatotoxicity) are noted in fewer than 2 percent of patients. Most liver abnormalities develop during the first three months of drug therapy, and are almost always reversible. We monitor our patients' liver function tests frequently during the initial stages of drug therapy to avoid significant liver problems down the line. Another side effect is rhabdomyolysis, a breakdown of skeletal muscles, which occurs in approximately 1 of every 1,000 patients taking this medication. This complication occurs more frequently when patients on statins add erythromycin or niacin to their drug regimen. Again, of all the cholesterol-lowering drugs, statins are the most effective at lowering LDL levels. When given with caution and care, these drugs can be valuable life-saving additions to our pharmaceutical armamentarium. Please remember, though, that they are not the answer to the problem of coronary artery disease; they are merely a piece of the puzzle and should be used when only absolutely necessary. If given the option of eating an unhealthful diet and taking a statin versus eating a good diet, taking various nutritional and vitamin supplements, and lowering cholesterol to appropriate levels while not taking a statin, the latter is clearly the better option.

Fibric Acid Derivatives

The fibric acid derivatives are a group of drugs only rarely used in managing cholesterol. They are often prescribed for patients with extremely high triglycerides (a blood test level greater than 400) that cannot be managed with dietary intervention and essential fatty acids. Gemfibrozil is the most commonly utilized drug in this class, and although poorly understood in terms of its action, can reduce VLDL (very low density lipoproteins) by 20–50 percent of baseline levels.

Other side benefits involve an HDL increase of 10–15 percent, a reduction in platelet aggregability, and a reduction in PAI-1, as is seen with the statins. Side effects are generally mild and may include gastrointestinal upset.

Estrogen Replacement Therapy

Estrogen replacement therapy (ERT) is a controversial area, not only for preventing osteoporosis, but also in preventing coronary disease. And as it is controversial, I do advise caution when deciding to use or not to use ERT. It is clear, though, that when women go through menopause and estrogen levels decrease, LDL and triglycerides increase while HDL falls. It is not clear, however, that the changes in these fat components are due solely to changes in estrogen levels, since progesterone levels also change significantly during menopause. It is still unclear whether estrogen replacement improves cardiovascular morbidity and mortality in postmenopausal women. One study, for example, has demonstrated clear efficacy of estrogen here. Giving women only estrogen—called "unopposed estrogen"—is also associated with increases in breast and endometrial

TABLE 5
Medications That Help to Prevent Coronary Artery Disease by Lowering High LDL Cholesterol Levels

Drug	Action	Potential Side Effects
Statins (HMG-CoA reductase inhibitors): Mevacor Pravachol Zocor Lipitor	Most effective; can decrease LDL levels by 20–40%. Statins increase liver LDL receptors, thereby lowering the amount of LDL circulating in the blood.	• Liver toxicity. • Can interact with niacin or erythromycin to produce muscle fiber breakdown.
Fibric acid derivatives: Lopid	Lowers triglycerides as much as 20–50%, and may increase HDL cholesterol as much as 10–15%. It's not understood how these drugs work.	• Mild GI upset.
Estrogen replacement therapy	Appears to counteract post-menopausal changes, keeping LDL and triglycerides from increasing and HDL from decreasing.	• Potential increase in risk of developing breast and/or endometrial cancer. • Can increase triglyceride levels.

cancers, something we don't want to cause! With the addition of progesterone, however, the risk of developing these cancers falls, and lipid benefits seem to be maintained. You should know that oral estrogen therapy is more effective than "the patch" (transcutaneous therapy). You should also know that ERT is one of the causes of elevated triglyceride levels, revealing estrogen as having both a positive *and* a negative effect on our bodies' fat components.

Interestingly enough, in the Coronary Artery Drug Project study, researchers evaluated 8,300 *men* with prior myocardial infarctions in relation to ERT. The men were divided into two groups and given dosages of ERT. In each of these treatment groups, the men taking estrogen had an increase in nonfatal heart attacks and in cardiovascular mortality, cancer mortality, and blood clots (or thromboembolic events). Thus, ERT is certainly not advocated for men and is still under significant review for postmenopausal women.

Now that we have reviewed the evaluative studies on cholesterol lowering, the drugs used to achieve cholesterol lowering, and the cardiovascular morbidity and mortality reductions they provide, we must look at why cholesterol can damage arteries, and how low is too low for cholesterol.

Cholesterol: The Good, the Bad, and the Necessary

As I stated earlier, cholesterol is vital in maintaining our bodies' health. In fact, without adequate amounts of cholesterol, our cell membranes would be less pliable, our nerve tissue less functional, and our bodies' steroid synthesis impaired. LDL is the form of cholesterol that delivers fats to all these tissues. Why, then, is LDL cholesterol bad? Well, it appears that it is not LDL, per se, that is bad but only its oxidized form. Oxidized LDL can attract circulating white blood cells (monocytes) from within our blood. They, in turn, become "aggressive," adhering to arterial walls and penetrating them. As monocytes enter the blood vessel walls, they become macrophages. Later, laden with oxidized LDL, these macrophages contribute to the buildup of an atherosclerotic plaque. Thus, we wish to limit not just the amount of LDL in our bloodstream, but the *oxidation* of LDL. That's why we so often recommend antioxidants like vitamin E, alpha lipoic acid, vitamin C, and grape seed extract to combat heart disease.

How low should we get our cholesterol levels, and is there a level that is too low? Let's look at the guidelines of cholesterol-lowering therapy as outlined by the National Cholesterol Education Program (NCEP), a panel associated with the National Institutes of Health. The NCEP advises that children ages 2 to 19 years be screened when they have a family history of premature atherosclerotic heart disease or hypercholesterolemia. If their LDL is 170 or greater, a cholesterol-lowering diet is recommended. If the LDL cholesterol remains over 190 after one year of good dietary management, or if it remains over 160 and the patient has either a family history of coronary disease or two other cardiac risk factors, then cholesterol-lowering drugs are recommended (as long as the patient is over 10 years of age).

NCEP guidelines are different in adults. If the LDL is over 190, regardless of a patient's risk factors, cholesterol-lowering drugs are recommended. When the LDL is over 160 in a patient with greater than two risk factors, drugs are recommended; and if the LDL is over 130 and the patient has documented coronary disease, again drugs are recommended. We generally like patients with documented coronary artery disease to have LDL levels under 100. Of course, dietary management is recommended by the NCEP, but if diet is inadequate, drug therapy, following the guidelines just outlined, is also recommended. Don't forget, however, that herbal and fiber supplements can often be used to achieve excellent cholesterol lowering without using pharmaceutical agents. When supplements fail, however, drugs should be administered, as advised by the NCEP.

Because of our aggressive pursuit of low cholesterol levels, there are concerns that cholesterol levels that are too low can lead to illness and even death—epidemiologic studies have revealed an increase in mortality in patients with extremely low cholesterol levels. This is a dangerously misleading statistic. Cholesterol falls precipitously when patients have severe underlying diseases such as cancers, lung disease, and cirrhosis. It is, therefore, unclear that the studies revealing a relationship between low cholesterol and an increased risk of untimely death have, in fact, demonstrated cause and effect.

There is other, additional evidence that low cholesterol levels do *not* predispose a person to increased mortality. For instance, a study of Shanghai citizens demonstrated a mean cholesterol level of 162 without any increase in the risk of cancer or other deaths. A disease called A-betalipoproteinemia, in which cholesterol levels are between 20 and 40, carries with it no increased risk of mortality. These patients suffer from peripheral neuropathies due to the low fat content in their nerves, but they do not have any increased risk of dying. Thus, I feel comfortable that, at the level of cholesterol lowering achieved through drug management, we are not jeopardizing our patients or subjecting them to an increased risk of dying.

Most of our discussion so far has focused on LDL and its effect on cardiovascular mortality. Many patients have elevations in triglyceride levels and are concerned that this, too, may portend an increased risk of cardiovascular mortality. However, there is still a question about whether hypertriglyceridemia predisposes to coronary artery disease but it seems that it probably does. A large "meta-analysis" of over 38,000 patients demonstrated an increased risk of cardiovascular disease in patients with elevated triglycerides. It is generally felt that triglyceride levels between 200 and 300 are the most damaging to our coronary arteries.

There are many causes of high triglycerides that can be effectively dealt with prior to using drug therapy. These include diabetes; hypothyroidism (low thyroid); obesity; the use of certain drugs, including beta blockers, diuretics, and estrogen replacement therapy; high-carbohydrate diets; a high intake of alcohol; and a low intake of fat.

After addressing these potential causes of elevated triglycerides, my preferred therapy is a natural one: the use of the omega-3 fatty acids DHA and EPA. Although not yet recommended by the NCEP, I have found these fatty acids to be extremely effective at lowering triglycerides in my clinical practice. There is also evidence that increasing consumption of these omega-3 fatty acids may reduce the risk of cardiovascular disease. In fact, in a study of the Greenland Eskimos, along with the MRFIT trials, researchers demonstrated that cardiovascular disease is inversely proportional to the consumption of omega-3 fatty acids. A high intake of these omega-3 fatty acids decreases VLDL and also increases the best form of HDL (HDL-2). Studies have also shown that a higher intake of the omega-3 fatty acids results in lower blood pressure readings. I have found this to be true in my own practice, too. Thus, supplementation with the omega-3 fatty acids, or significantly increasing the consumption of cold water fish (such as salmon and mackerel), leads to improvements in triglyceride levels, blood pressure readings, and also most likely decreases the risk of developing future cardiovascular events.

Modifiable Causes of High Triglycerides

Alcohol intake
Diet (too much carbohydrate and too little fat)
Diabetes
Obesity
Low thyroid
Drugs (beta blockers, diuretics, and estrogen replacement therapy)

It's also important to understand LPa's role in coronary artery disease, even though the NCEP does not currently recommend routine measurements of LPa. LPa (an abbreviation for "lipoprotein a") has been found to be an independent risk factor for coronary artery disease. Its structure is nearly identical to that of LDL. In fact, LPa has been described as a particularly sticky form of LDL, which tends to adhere more readily to the endothelium of our blood vessels. LPa is also thought to be much more susceptible to oxidation than "regular" LDL and, thus potentially plays a more aggressive role in the creation of coronary disease.

As I mentioned earlier, taking niacin is the best means of lowering LPa levels. We need not concern ourselves too much with LPa, however, as long as we are able to achieve low LDL levels—LPa appears to lose its significance when LDL levels are effectively lowered. Even so, when patients have only mildly elevated LDL levels and extremely elevated LPa levels, I advocate the use of niacin.

Tobacco

Cigarette smoking is a hideous habit which unquestionably causes coronary artery disease. My 9-year-old son loves to quote the statistic that "every cigarette smoked leads to a five-minute loss of life." At his young age, he is fortunate enough to understand that smoking kills. Sadly, 46 million adult Americans do not understand what my 9-year-old does. Consequently, over 400,000 Americans die annually as a direct result of using tobacco. The Framingham study demonstrated an increase in cardiovascular mortality of 18 percent in men and 31 percent in women for every ten cigarettes smoked per day. Yes, *every* cigarette counts. Nor is just the inhalation of large quantities of smoke that kills, but the inhalation of any smoke that is important. Additionally, those of us who don't smoke but are simply exposed to cigarette smoke also experience a significant increase in our risk of cardiovascular mortality. In fact, 40,000 deaths a year are attributed to the effects of secondhand smoke. Amazingly, even smokeless tobacco results in an increased risk of cardiovascular death.

A common fallacy propagated through clever marketing is that low-tar cigarettes are safer than others. Tobacco companies often suggest that using their low-tar tobacco can decrease the cardiovascular risk of smoking. This is not true. Low-tar tobacco does not decrease the risk of coronary disease. The only way to eliminate the dangers of tobacco is to stop smoking.

Quitting smoking has clearly been shown to decrease the risk of cardiovascular disease, peripheral vascular disease, lung cancer, and chronic lung disease. It also improves one's cholesterol profile by raising HDL and lowering LDL, and it decreases platelet aggregability. Some studies have shown a slight increase in diastolic blood pressure as a result of smoking cessation, but this has been attributed to the weight gain that often occurs when people quit smoking. Still, the benefits of smoking cessation grossly outweigh the risks of the slight weight gain that can occur when breaking this awful habit.

It's tragic that only 50 percent of smokers are encouraged to quit smoking by their health care professionals. Obviously we doctors and nurses must do much more in our fight against tobacco.

Hypertension

Forty-three million Americans are known to suffer from hypertension (high blood pressure). Often called "the silent killer," high blood pressure usually has no symptoms. It is thus imperative that people have regular checkups with their physicians to ensure that they are not harboring this quiet but deadly disease. As we age, hypertension increases in frequency. Numerous studies also show that elevated blood pressure leads to the development of coronary artery and cerebrovascular disease (strokes). In a meta-analysis of over 400,000 patients evaluated in nine prospective studies, a clear correlation between blood pressure levels and the development of both coronary and cerebrovascular disease was found. In fact, for each 7.5 mm elevation of diastolic blood pressure, there was a 29 percent increase in the risk of cardiovascular disease.

TABLE 6
Lifestyle Changes That May Help to Prevent Coronary Artery Disease by Lowering High Blood Pressure

- Control obesity.
- Diminish alcohol intake.
- Eliminate cigarettes.
- Exercise regularly.

TABLE 6 (Continued)
Lifestyle Changes That May Help to Prevent Coronary Artery Disease by Lowering High Blood Pressure

- Employ stress reduction techniques such as meditation, yoga, T'ai Chi, and others.
- Make dietary changes such as adding significantly increased amounts of high-fiber and potassium-rich foods (i.e., vegetables and fruits such as bananas and oranges) to your diet.

My own approach to hypertension includes the following: When a patient's blood pressure is dangerously high, I immediately prescribe a strong pharmaceutical agent. I also suggest herbs such as hawthorn, coleus forskohii, and khella, as well as other supplements such as magnesium, coenzyme Q-10, fiber, and a variety of antioxidants. Our nutritionist will help the patient maintain a diet promoting blood pressure reduction (i.e., a low-salt, high-potassium diet including lots of vegetables and cold water fish, plenty of fiber, and avoiding red meat). Over time as the patient's blood pressure falls adequately, the pharmaceuticals will be withdrawn, leaving the patient free from their potentially toxic side effects. I have found this approach extremely effective in a great number of hypertension patients. In those patients who have only mildly elevated blood pressure, I begin with a strictly natural approach, one free of drugs. If the natural approach fails to lower the blood pressure adequately, only then will I add drugs to the patient's regimen.

Table 7 lists the group supplements I use in helping patients to lower their blood pressure.

TABLE 7
Supplements That May Help Prevent Coronary Artery Disease by Lowering High Blood Pressure

Supplement	Recommended Daily Dosage
Garlic	4 mg of allicin potential
Magnesium	An extra 200 to 400 mg
Coleus forskohii	50 mg of an 18% forskolin standardized extract three times daily
Coenzyme Q-10	100 mg twice a day

TABLE 7 (Continued)
Supplements That May Help Prevent Coronary Artery Disease by Lowering High Blood Pressure

Calcium	In salt-sensitive people: an additional 500 mg
Khella extract	100 mg of a 12% khellin extract twice a day
Hawthorn	160 to 900 mg of leaf and flower extract in two divided doses
Omega-3 fatty acids	3 g of DHA and EPA (combined) in two divided doses
Fresh ginger	With meals, as frequently as possible
Garlic and onions	With meals, as frequently as possible
L-taurine	1.5 g twice a day on an empty stomach

Diabetes

Although not as common as hypertension, diabetes mellitus is still a major risk factor for coronary disease. Of the 14 million Americans who suffer from this ailment, almost all have non-insulin-dependent (Type 2) diabetes mellitus.

This is a disorder that increases with age, dietary indiscretion, and obesity. Of course, diabetes can affect all parts of the body, but it is vascular disease that is the most merciless killer of diabetics. Almost 80 percent of all American diabetics will die from vascular disease. The blood vessels serving any part of the body can be affected—and therefore, the kidneys, the eyes, the brain, the heart, and the legs can be destroyed by diabetes. Diabetics also often have elevated triglyceride levels and low HDL levels. Worse still, their LDL is more easily oxidized than "normal" LDL, making it a potent enemy of their arteries.

Despite all this, there is some controversy about the importance of controlling blood sugar in the diabetic population. This is because nearly 25 percent of all diabetics will not develop vascular complications regardless of their glucose control. Nevertheless, numerous studies show that diabetics can decrease eye disease (diabetic retinopathy), lipid abnormalities, and even death from cardiovascular disease when they do control their glucose. Thus, it is my feeling and that of the general medical community that controlling a patient's glucose is paramount in the management of diabetes mellitus.

Believe it or not, rigorous dietary changes alone will stabilize blood sugar levels in most adult-onset diabetes patients. According to David Levinson, M.D., a brilliant endocrinologist in Boca Raton, however, the problem is that many people find it easier to inject insulin than to alter their diet. This is hard to believe, but true. In addition, fiber supplements, chromium, coenzyme Q-10, and exercise will help to reduce blood sugar levels in diabetic patients.

Obesity

With 58 million adult Americans now defined as being obese, the condition has just recently been upgraded to a major cardiovascular risk factor. Of all obesities, central obesity—a condition in which excessive fat resides in the midportion of our body—is the most malevolent. One of the best trials demonstrating the influence of obesity on cardiovascular health was the Framingham Study, which clearly established obesity as an independent risk factor for coronary disease in both men and women.

It has also been shown that multiple episodes of weight loss and gain, the so-called yo-yo effect, increase the risk of future cardiovascular disease. In some instances, it may be better to remain overweight rather than continually lose and regain one's weight—but this is a decision that should be made in consultation with your physician. Obesity is a modifiable risk factor which should be addressed aggressively in order to limit the development of coronary artery disease. In Chapter 10, "If Chicken Soup is Penicillin, Then What Is This I'm Eating?," I'll explain several appropriate dietary strategies for weight management and health promotion.

Physical Inactivity

Sixty percent of all Americans are considered to be sedentary—a risk factor with substantial implications. We well know how exercise decreases your chance of developing cardiovascular disease. In fact, exercise increases HDL, improves insulin resistance, decreases blood pressure, decreases body weight, as well as benefiting your outlook. People who exercise regularly feel more relaxed and calmer. An avid exerciser will tell you that on days when he or she is unable to exercise, his or her anxiety level skyrockets. In Chapter 13, I will explore the various forms of exercise that can help you achieve better physical and emotional balance.

Type A Behavior Pattern

Emotions, being so subjective, are a notoriously difficult area to evaluate, especially in regard to their impact on health and disease. In fact, during my residency, I recall being told that stress plays no part whatsoever in the development of coronary disease. I have since grown to believe that stress plays a major role in the development of coronary disease as well as in other disease processes. Indeed, stress is deadly. It elevates levels of circulating substances such as epinephrine, norepinephrine, and cortisol which, when chronically elevated, can have devastating effects on our bodies. In examining stress in relationship to coronary artery disease, the most commonly employed model is the "type A personality" or "behavior pattern." As we know, the "type A personality" is high strung, given to constant anxiety, and suffers the effects of stress all too much.

The Western Collaborative Group Study is a particularly important piece of research on type A behavior patterns. It demonstates a two-fold increase in the development of coronary disease in patients who exhibit the behavior we associate with type A. The Framingham Study also revealed a twofold increase in angina with type A behavior patterns, but no increase in heart attack or death. Interestingly, several studies have demonstrated increased cardiovascular risk in people prone to excessive worry or anxiety, and who make no attempt to stay calm during minor altercations. Be that as it may, the MRFIT trial did not demonstrate any increased risk for cardiac events in patients with type A behavior pattern. In my view, however, I believe stress is extremely important. And when I encounter stress in a patient, whether he or she is "type A" or not, I always offer regimens to reduce it, including supplements, medication, exercise, and stress-reduction programs.

Low Level of Circulating Antioxidants

In the battle against coronary disease, much attention has been paid recently to antioxidants. Studies show that low levels of antioxidants increase the risk of cardiovascular events. Vitamin E supplementation, for example, has proved therapeutic in this regard. And how does this happen? Antioxidants *reduce* the susceptibility of LDLs and LPa's to oxidative injury, itself a main cause of their detrimental effects on coronary arteries. I, therefore, urge that all my patients take adequate quantities of antioxidants, including vitamins C and E, alpha lipoic acid, coenzyme Q-10, and grape seed extract.

Blood Factors

Several components of our blood—PAI-1, factor 7, fibrinogen, homocysteine, and even iron—have all been found to be risk factors for coronary artery disease when present in "inappropriate" amounts. Although there currently is no formal recommendation for altering the levels of these substances, they still bear mentioning.

Plasminogen Activator Inhibitor 1 (PAI-1)

Earlier in this chapter, we discussed plasminogen activator inhibitor 1 (PAI-1). When PAI-1 levels are elevated, a decrease in fibrinolytic activity may ensue, which means that one's blood might clot more readily. Gemfibrozil and the statins decrease PAI-1, thus potentially lessening cardiovascular risk. Please note that, in the absense of studies sufficient to determine clinical relevance, doctors do not usually monitor PAI-1 levels.

Factor 7

Factor 7, one of our clotting factors, has been shown to increase the frequency of coronary artery disease in several epidemiologic studies. This factor may have particular importance because an increase in dietary consumption of fat results in an increase in Factor 7, and thus may predispose a person to coronary artery disease. This is just another example of why paying close attention to our dietary fat may help save our lives.

Fibrinogen

An elevated level of fibrinogen, another blood component that helps promote clotting, is another risk factor for cardiovascular disease. When comparing Americans and Japanese, scientists have found that Americans have much higher levels of fibrinogen than do Japanese. This may help explain why the Japanese have a much lower incidence of coronary disease. It has not yet been scientifically established, but perhaps the Japanese diet is responsible for a lower level of fibrinogen, thus leading to a diminished frequency of heart disease.

Homocysteine

Homocysteine is produced by protein metabolism. Recently, homocysteine has become a household word, as Dr. Kilmer McCulley's work, which he performed at Harvard in the 1970s, has finally become popularized. Dr. McCulley was the first to recognize the correlation between elevated homocysteine levels and coronary artery disease. He also noted that vitamins B_6, B_{12}, and folic acid help reduce homocysteine levels and thus might help prevent future coronary events. Because of his novel and natural approach to disease, Dr. McCulley and his theory were not exactly welcomed with open arms by the medical community. Unfortunately this is *not* an uncommon scenario. (On a smaller scale, I have experienced a similar professional ostracism.) As a result, only recently has Dr. McCulley's theory gained the recognition it deserves. Now there are numerous ongoing studies examining the impact of homocysteine and homocysteine lowering in coronary artery disease patients. In my personal practice, I have been measuring homocysteine levels for over two years and have found monitoring them to be extremely beneficial in helping to reduce cardiovascular risks. In the majority of my patients as well, vitamins B_6, B_{12}, and folic acid have been extremely effective in lowering homocysteine levels.

Iron

Iron is a mineral of growing concern to cardiovascular researchers. In fact, there are some studies that point to elevated levels of iron as damaging to coronary arteries. The reason is more of a hypothesis at this stage, but it's one that allopathic and alternative medical professionals are aware of. Simply, iron may act as a free radical, wreaking havoc on our arterial linings. A corollary of this theory is that premenopausal women have less coronary disease precisely because of their iron deficiency (a result of menstrual bleeding). Given these and other considerations, in my practice I keep a keen eye on iron intake whether by diet or supplementation.

CHAPTER 5

The Pipes Are Clogged

Let's now look at the many faces of coronary disease and detail the treatment options currently available.

Certainly, coronary artery disease represents a spectrum of disorders, ranging from the patient with occasional chest pain (chronic, stable angina pectoris) to the patient enduring a major heart attack (acute myocardial infarction). We'll visit each of the major pit stops along the road of atherosclerotic heart disease.

Chronic Stable Angina Pectoris

What is chronic stable angina? "Chronic" implies that a condition is long-standing. Stable, of course, implies that a condition is relatively safe, meaning that there is a low likelihood of a dramatic and terrible event occurring in the not-too-distant future. "Angina" refers to a type of discomfort associated with coronary artery disease. The classic manifestation of anginal pain is a squeezing, pressure-like sensation in the mid-sternum (that is, the mid-portion of the chest). The pain can radiate to the neck, the jaw, the left arm, or even the right arm. At times, this tightness moves to the back; at other times it moves to the belly. Its typical form, however, is in the chest, which is why it's referred to as angina pectoris ("pectoris" is Latin for "chest").

Because there are so many atypical forms of this type of discomfort, actually diagnosing it as angina can often be difficult both for patients and physicians. I have had patients in my practice, for example, whose only manifestation of angina was a pain in the wrist, in the belly, in the teeth, or simply mild shortness of breath with exertion.

Of even greater concern are those patients with no symptoms at all and yet who suffer from significant coronary arterial blockage. These patients have "silent ischemia," and are at a higher risk of developing acute events (like heart attacks) because of their absence of symptoms. Generally, cardiologists feel that they should treat these patients very aggressively, performing coronary interventions when indicated (usually by abnormal stress test results).

Symptoms of Angina Pectoris

- "Squeezing" pressure in the chest
- Tightness or pain radiating from the chest to the neck, jaw, or either arm
- Tightness in the back
- Pain in the teeth
- Unusual: tightness or pain in the wrist, belly, or teeth
- Mild shortness of breath on exertion (not always a symptom of angina)

As you can see, angina pectoris has a variety of manifestations, which can make for some confusion. Other conditions that can be mistaken for angina pectoris include esophageal disorders (such as esophageal spasm or reflux esophagitis), gallbladder disease, neck problems, inflammation of the rib cartilage, and inflammation of the lining of the heart.

When receiving a diagnosis of chronic stable angina pectoris, one should know this: In itself, it connotes a relatively low-risk condition, even though the symptoms can be scary. In fact, there is only about a 1–2 percent annual incidence of heart attacks (myocardial infarctions) here.

Possibly because of the inherent low risk in this group of patients, it is difficult to demonstrate long-term benefits derived from drug treatments. Interestingly, among the many medicines used for treating chronic stable angina, only aspirin and the cholesterol-lowering medicines have been shown to decrease morbidity and mortality. In a meta-analysis which evaluated 140,000 patients taking aspirin in over 500 studies, a clear prophylactic benefit was derived in both men and women with prior heart attacks, angina pectoris, prior strokes, or a history of coronary artery bypass grafting. Although there is still debate about what dose of aspirin best decreases cardiovascular risks, one baby aspirin a day, perhaps supplemented with one 325 mg aspirin every two weeks, is a reasonable recommendation.

Many other medications—including drugs like Coumadin (a blood thinner), the angiotensin converting enzyme inhibitors, and the beta blockers—which have been evaluated in chronic stable angina, have proved less successful with no significant benefit in reducing mortality. Nevertheless, if a patient has had a prior heart attack, beta blockers decrease future cardiovascular events, and the angiotensin converting enzyme inhibitors diminish future cardiovascular problems in patients with documented coronary disease and weakened heart muscles.

The medical management of coronary artery disease, according to Eugene Braunwald (as explained in his *Textbook of Cardiovascular Medicine*), includes four components, and each must be satisfied for every patient.

- First, the doctor must identify and treat any associated diseases which may either precipitate or worsen angina, such as anemia or increased thyroid hormone levels.
- Next, the physician must diminish cardiovascular risks, as we discussed in Chapter 4. This should include lifestyle changes which, although difficult at times to implement, can truly be life-saving. In Chapter 6, we'll examine the important lifestyle changes that must be made, and ways to begin to make them.
- Pharmacologic therapy is another component of the treatment of coronary artery disease, and we'll discuss it in great detail later in the chapter.
- The fourth component is revascularization—that is, employing procedures that improve coronary anatomy (usually either angioplasty or bypass surgery). These, too, will be extensively examined later in this chapter.

Let's first examine the drugs that are the mainstay of current traditional medical therapy for angina and then turn to natural preparations. Three categories of drugs are utilized by most cardiologists in the management of chronic, stable angina pectoris: nitrates, beta blockers, and calcium channel blockers.

Nitrates

Nitroglycerine is an immensely effective medication for relieving angina pectoris. When patients experience episodes of angina, we often advise them to take small tablets of nitroglycerine under their tongues or to spray nitroglycerine in their mouths for prompt relief. Nitrates date back many years in the management of coronary disease, with the first clinical use of amyl nitrite in 1867.

Since then, a whole series of diverse forms of nitrates, from short-acting to long-acting, have been developed. These agents act through various means. They help relax vascular smooth muscle, producing an effect not just on the coronary arteries but also on the vessels in our arms, legs, and the rest of our body. By relaxing these vessels, nitrates relieve the burden on the heart, in turn diminishing the heart's need for its blood supply and oxygen. By making the heart's job easier, nitroglycerine reduces angina.

An interesting and little-known fact is that the effect of nitrates is not limited to vascular dilation. Nitroglycerine is also endowed with the heart-protective anticlotting (antithrombotic) effect of blocking platelet aggregation.

Since hundreds of thousands of people in America rely on nitrates to treat their angina, it is important to realize that patients can actually become "tolerant" to their nitroglycerine. Patients who take nitroglycerine too frequently, thus maintaining continuously elevated blood levels of the substance, can also forfeit its benefits. To avoid this pitfall, the body must be free of nitrates for at least ten to twelve hours a day. The body needs this time to metabolize nitroglycerine properly. This is why we tell our patients to remove their nitroglycerine patches after twelve hours of use, and why most doctors prefer once-a-day nitroglycerine preparations.

You may find it interesting to note that nitric oxide is the powerful substance released by Viagra that allows this anti-impotence drug to do its work. The side effects of nitrates and Viagra are similar, usually limited in duration, and can include headaches, flushing, and sometimes a significant drop in blood pressure. When patients develop headaches as a result, we generally advise them to take Tylenol rather than aspirin, so as to save them possible upset stomach or even ulcers.

Beta Blockers

Beta blockers are very effective agents for treating chronic stable angina. Like nitrates, they diminish the heart's need for oxygen consumption, thus lessening its need for blood flow. They perform this vital task by decreasing heart rate, blood pressure, and the heart's ability to squeeze vigorously (called "inotropy"). These three changes enable the heart to function at a level that requires less blood flow, thus allowing it to compensate for blocked arteries.

Our main goal with beta blocker therapy is to lower the patient's resting heart rate (i.e., the heart rate when sitting down) to 50–60 beats per minute, compared to a "normal" resting heart beat of 60–100. The "beta blocked" patient will also have far less of an elevation in heart rate when performing mild exercise, compared to a person not taking beta blockers.

While these drugs are extremely effective at decreasing angina, they do, at times, cause side effects. Most cardiologists, for example, are concerned that beta blockers generally increase triglycerides and decrease the protective component of cholesterol, HDL. You should also be concerned about any agent that decreases the heart-protective HDL. Another potential side effect is a constriction of the bronchi (the small tubules in the lungs that normally allow us to breathe easily), particularly in patients with asthma. Thus, beta blockers can occasionally precipitate asthma attacks. Depression, fatigue, nightmares, and hair loss are other side effects of several of the beta blockers. At times, patients develop cold extremities, and those with blockages in arteries feeding the legs can develop leg pain while using beta blockers.

For patients taking beta blockers, it is crucial that they do not abruptly stop taking them. You can't run out of a beta blocker prescription on Friday and wait until Monday to fill it. Patients who do this often end up with a rapid and frightening progression in their angina pectoris.

TABLE 8
Medications Used to Treat Angina Pectoris

Drug	Action	Potential Side Effects
Aspirin	May reduce angina in people with prior heart attacks, angina pectoris, prior strokes, or history of bypass surgery. It definitely reduces heart attacks.	• Easy bruising may occur. • Can irritate the lining of the gastrointestinal system.
Nitrates: Sublingual nitroglycerine, Imdur, transdermal nitroglycerine	Stop angina by relaxing vascular smooth muscle, making the heart's job easier. Can also block blood clot formation.	• Overuse can result in tolerance, so the medication stops working. • Headache. • Flushing. • Drop in blood pressure.
Beta Blockers: Tenormin, Lopressor	Diminish the heart's need for oxygen (like the nitrates) by decreasing heart rate and blood pressure, and making the heart muscle work less hard.	• Can increase triglycerides. • Can decrease heart-protective HDL cholesterol. • Can cause difficulty breathing and precipitate asthma attacks. • Can cause leg pain or sensitivity to cold in patients whose arteries in the legs are blocked. • Hair loss. • Depression. • Fatigue. • Nightmares.
Calcium channel blockers such as nifedipine	Of the calcium channel blockers they have the greatest effect on expanding blood vessels. They have minimal effect on heart muscle function and heart rate.	• Headaches. • Palpitations. Flushing. • Dizziness. • Swelling of legs. • Gastrointestinal problems. • Short-acting versions may contribute to mortality in patients with heart disease.
Calcium channel blockers such as diltiazem	These drugs decrease heart rate and strength of contractility. They also expand blood vessels.	• Headaches. • Constipation. • Flushing. • Gum swelling.

TABLE 8 (Continued)
Medications Used to Treat Angina Pectoris

Drug	Action	Potential Side Effects
Calcium channel blockers such as verapamil	Of the calcium channel blockers, these drugs have the greatest effect on slowing the heart rate and decreasing contractility.	• Headaches. • Constipation. • Flushing. • Dizziness. • Palpitations. • Gastrointestinal problems.

Thus, while beta blockers are extremely beneficial in managing coronary artery disease, they must be used cautiously and conscientiously, and patients should be aware of their potential side effects.

Calcium Channel Blockers

Although the calcium channel blockers form a heterogeneous group of drugs, they are still generally lumped together. The three major groups of calcium channel blockers are exemplified by three drugs: nifedipine, diltiazem, and verapamil. On one end of the spectrum lies nifedipine and other drugs of its class. On the other end is verapamil and its cousins. In the middle lies diltiazem and the other drugs that resemble it.

Drugs such as nifedipine act predominantly as vasodilators, meaning they expand blood vessels. They have little effect on heart rate or on inotropy (the squeeze of the heart). Their most common side effects include headaches, palpitations, flushing, dizziness, and swelling of the lower extremities. Occasionally, some patients develop gastrointestinal difficulty. Recent studies of the short-acting form of nifedipine showed that it may increase mortality in cardiovascular patients, and thus generated bad press for all of the calcium channel blockers. Be that as it may, there is no clear evidence that either the other calcium channel blockers or the longer-acting ones will exhibit this detrimental effect. It was found only in short-acting nifedipine.

Verapamil's action is almost exactly opposite to nifedipine's: Verapamil very significantly decreases heart rate. Verapamil also possesses a strongly negative effect on the heart's ability to squeeze forcefully (inotropy). Side effects of verapamil include headaches, constipation, flushing, and a swelling of the gums (referred to as "gingival hyperplasia").

Diltiazem and other drugs of its category have effects lying between those of nifedipine and verapamil. They slow the heart rate to some extent, they decrease inotropy to some extent, and they vasodilate more prominently than verapamil. Side effects of these drugs are similar to those of verapamil and nifedipine.

All classes of calcium channel blockers are used frequently by cardiologists, not just to treat angina pectoris but also to manage hypertension.

Let's also not forget the natural remedies useful in treating angina (see Table 9). Hawthorn and khella, herbs that act as vasodilators, have been shown to possess significant utility in managing this type of chest pain. L-carnitine and coenzyme Q-10, augmenting the heart's ability to create energy, have also aided patients suffering from this disorder. Antioxidant vitamins such as C and E are very useful in treating angina patients. Interestingly, bromelain (an enzyme extracted from pineapples) has also been reported to limit the frequency of chest pain when taken on an empty stomach by angina patients. Of course, this does not mean that you should throw away your nitroglycerine and replace it with hawthorn. Please discuss all herbal and medication changes with your doctor prior to making them. Keeping your doctor informed will definitely help to improve your health.

Unfortunately, drug therapy and natural remedies are not always completely effective in treating chronic stable angina, and more aggressive approaches sometimes must be used. Invasive techniques such as angioplasty and coronary artery bypass surgery, however, have both benefits and drawbacks for patients. Let's look at some of them now.

Remember this though: If you or a loved one require angioplasty or surgery be sure to find a surgeon with much experience in the procedure—statistics show that their success rate is higher than other less experienced surgeons.

Interventional Cardiology

First, what is interventional cardiology? It is a subspecialty in which physicians snake catheters, wires, and other devices into the

TABLE 9
Natural Preparations Used to Treat Angina Pectoris

Supplement	Recommended Daily Dosage
Hawthorn extract	160 to 900 mg of flower and leaf (preferred), standardized to 10% procyanidin content, in two divided doses
Khella extract	100 mg of 12% khellin three times daily
L-carnitine	1 g, twice daily
Bromelain	150 to 500 mg three times daily on an empty stomach
Omega-3 fatty acids	3 g DHA and EPA (combined) daily
Vitamin E	400–800 IU daily
Vitamin C	1,000–2,000 mg daily
Coenzyme Q-10	60–150 mg daily

arteries that feed the heart, via small punctures in various "peripheral" arteries and veins. During these procedures, patients are sedated but awake.

The first "balloon angioplasty" was performed in 1964. The doctors opened a blocked blood vessel that fed a patient's leg. There were so many complications with early angioplasty, however, that it was not pursued aggressively until the late 1970s. In 1977, in Zurich, Switzerland, Dr. Andreas Grunzig performed the first percutaneous transluminal coronary angioplasty (PTCA) on a 37-year-old man with angina pectoris. Since that success, the use of angioplasty has increased so dramatically that well over 400,000 are now performed annually in the United States alone.

To my knowledge, there is only one significant randomized trial which compared medical therapy (i.e., drugs) to angioplasty, the ACME (Angioplasty Compared to Medicine) trial. This study demonstrated that, when only one artery is clogged ("single vessel disease"), angioplasty produced better outcomes than medical therapy in decreasing symptoms of angina. No mortality benefit was demonstrated but angioplasty definitely alleviated symptoms.

Unfortunately, angioplasty has three notable limitations: First, many vessels cannot be approached with a balloon because of their tortuosity (extreme bends), heavy calcification, or small caliber. Second, a small subset of patients (2–5 percent) experience an abrupt closure of their vessel during PTCA. This can result in a heart attack, the need for an emergency coronary artery bypass grafting, or even death. Third, about 30–40 percent of patients undergoing simple balloon angioplasty develop restenosis, a disorder in which the arterial blockage returns within as little as six to eight months.

What are the new techniques recently developed to address these problems? The "drills," of course, are true to their name. In the earliest drill technique, called directional coronary atherectomy (DCA), a physician uses a cutting tool with a hollowed-out canoe containing a rotating blade which cuts the plaque and presses it into a nose cone. He or she can then remove the compressed plaque from the patient's body with ease.

When I began performing DCAs in the early 1990s, I, like many of my colleagues, was elated. Here was the perfect answer to all our problems. And, in fact, DCA is effective, especially in approaching complex blockages. Evaluation studies, however, did not show any

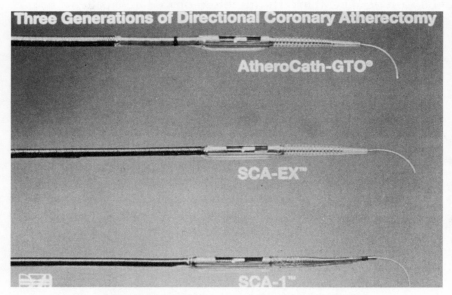

Three Generations of Directional Coronary Atherectomy

benefit over "plain old balloon angioplasty" ("POBA") in terms of restenosis, and so the procedure has fallen out of favor.

The next cutting tool, the transluminal extraction catheter (TEC), also uses a cutting blade, but rotates it more slowly than the DCA. You can think of TEC as a tiny vacuum cleaner which, when placed in an old vein graft or a blood vessel possessing clumps of clot, can actually suck material out of the body into small vials of fluid (the cardiologist's version of liposuction). Although this device opened up new areas for the interventional cardiologist, it did not lower the rate at which restenosis takes place.

The final cutting tool is called the "rotablator." A high-speed, conically shaped, diamond-coated burr, spinning at 80,000 revolutions per minute, the rotablator pulverizes tissue into tiny particles smaller than red blood cells. Although this device may sound frightening, it is fairly safe to use. In fact, it allows cardiologists to clear heavily calcified and tortuous vessels and even vessels of very small caliber. Of the three cutting devices, I prefer the rotablator as do most of my colleagues. Unfortunately, it also does not diminish restenosis.

The laser—a noncutting (but burning) device—was conceived to improve the outcome of angioplasty. Cardiologists were thrilled

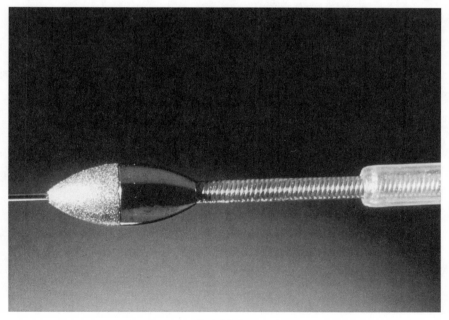

Rotablater

when the Excimer laser was released for clinical use. It conjured futuristic images of laser-wielding warriors of coronary disease. Unfortunately, the laser also proved to be ineffective and too risky for actual use. As a result, lasers are now used much more modestly to remove defective pacemaker wires.

The stent, which was created as a mechanical solution to restenosis, abrupt closure, and the limitations of angioplasty, consists of a small wire mesh that is permanently embedded in coronary arteries at blockage sites. Today, there are myriad stents, and they do appear to decrease restenosis to about 15–20 percent. In fact, stents are now so widely utilized that they have become the great equalizer for interventional cardiologists, enabling many such physicians to perform interventional procedures safely.

In Chapter 3, I told you about Martha Lee, who underwent nearly every cardiac test imaginable. She learned from these tests that her LAD coronary artery was clogged with a 90–95 percent proximal (at its origin) stenosis. Because of the severe nature of her blockage and her somewhat unstable presentation, Mrs. Lee underwent angio-

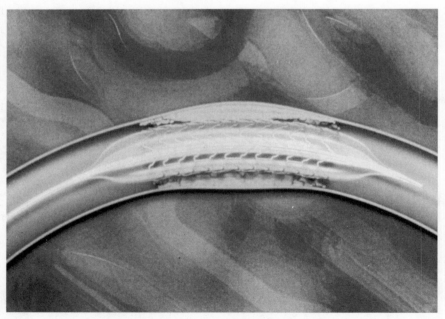

Stent on Balloon

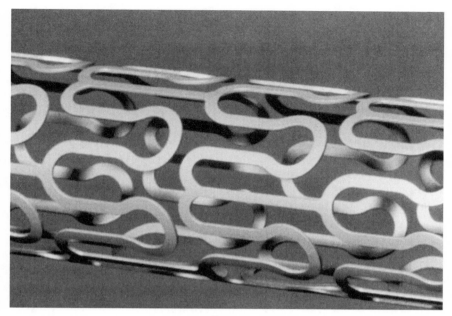

Stent

plasty (a PTCA) and stent placement. She had an excellent outcome, with a complete resolution of not only her obstruction, but also her symptoms. Mrs. Lee has since "changed her life." She walks daily, eats a diet rich in vegetables, fruits, and fish and low in saturated fats, and meditates every morning to reduce her stress. She's not only healthier but also much more relaxed.

Certainly, without the benefit of her stent, Mrs. Lee would have been unable to live an angina-free existence. She is one of the millions who have enjoyed the benefits of today's technology. Just as important, she is one of the intelligent few who understand the need to become an active participant in the process of achieving and maintaining health. Her *continuing* lifestyle changes will endow her with the greatest chances of *not* requiring future cardiovascular interventions.

In addition to all of the technological advances made in angioplasty, a pharmacologic advance in Reopro, a drug which limits the stickiness of platelets, has also proved effective at lowering restenosis rates and decreasing mortality. The only current drawback to this drug is its expense, costing as much as $1,000–$2,000 per patient per administration. Ongoing research, however, is studying the benefits of this and other types of antiplatelet agents. Hopefully, in the not-too-distant future, the price will fall as other competitive agents emerge.

Cornary Artery Bypass Grafting

Coronary artery bypass grafting (CABG, also often known as ACB or aortocoronary bypass) is the most aggressive therapy now available to manage chronic stable angina. During this surgical procedure, cardiothoracic surgeons open a patient's chest in order to attach new vessels beyond the areas of arterial blockage. By circumventing prior blockage, these new blood vessels, whether veins or arteries, allow adequate supplies of blood and oxygen to the heart muscle. The patient's own blocked blood vessels are not *replaced,* a common misconception among laypeople. They are simply *bypassed.*

The history of the first coronary artery bypass grafting is somewhat special. In 1964 Drs. Garrett, Dennis, and DeBakey at the University of Texas in Houston first performed the procedure as a "bailout" in an emergency attempt to save a patient's life. Nineteen years later, by 1983, surgeons were performing 100,000 bypasses annually, and by 1993 that number had tripled. Currently, surgeons perform 400,000–500,000 bypass surgeries annually in the United States.

Through the years, of course, surgeons have used different bypass conduits. The most frequently employed vessels are vein grafts, harvested from the legs and then transplanted to the heart. Because of the tendency for vein grafts to develop recurrent blockage, surgeons have explored using other vessels for grafting, including the mammary artery. The mammary arteries, both left and right, lie on the inside of the chest, providing blood and nourishment to the chest wall. A surgeon will often use only a single mammary artery during a bypass operation, usually the left internal mammary artery (LIMA) as a graft to the left anterior descending coronary artery.

At times, surgeons use both mammary arteries. Unfortunately, a small group of patients with bilateral mammary artery grafting develop a very serious complication in which the sternum actually dies because it's been deprived of blood. Infections within the chest cavity can result from this complication, and patients may require extensive surgery utilizing muscle flaps to reconstruct the destroyed chest wall. Because of this potential complication, many surgeons shy away from the use of bilateral mammary arteries, and instead combine a single mammary artery with multiple vein grafts.

My patients often ask why veins from the arms are not acceptable grafts for bypass surgery. Unfortunately, veins from the arms, which tend to close very rapidly, are not nearly so durable as vein grafts taken from legs. At times, though, a surgeon can use an *artery* from the arm, such as the radial artery, as an excellent bypass conduit.

What is it about arteries that makes them so much more valuable for grafting than veins? While veins tend to develop atherosclerosis fairly readily, arteries do not. In fact, by the end of the first year following bypass surgery, 15–20 percent of vein grafts are closed, and ten years after bypass, two-thirds of all vein grafts have closed. The mammary artery, on the other hand, which tends not to develop atherosclerosis, has a patency rate of around 90 percent at ten years, meaning that it's good for you and your heart for at least that amount of time. Other ways to help diminish the progressive blockage of vein grafts include the use of aspirin and aggressive cholesterol-lowering. Again, cholesterol can be lowered either naturally or with the help of drugs. My preference, when possible, is always a natural one. This, of course, requires active patient participation and an element of patience. It can take longer to lower cholesterol with herbs and diet, but it's worth the wait.

Interestingly, we are able to predict which specific grafts may close more readily than others. Grafts that feed arteries with less than a 50 percent blockage and grafts that feed very small arteries tend to close rather rapidly. This is why we do not bypass vessels with only mild or moderate blockage (i.e., less than 60–70 percent).

Recently, there has been some talk about the lack of "appropriateness" or "necessity" of many of the bypass operations performed in the United States. But is that the case? One study said no, finding only 4 percent of bypasses in New York and Canada as inappropriate. Other reports suggest a contrary conclusion, noting a much higher incidence of "inappropriate" bypass grafting. Obviously, there is significant subjectivity in determining the appropriateness or inappropriateness of this operation. To help clarify this issue, during the 1970s three major studies—the VA Cooperative Study, the European

Cooperative Surgical Study (ECSS), and the Coronary Artery Surgical Study (CASS)—were done. These studies predated the routine use of aspirin and the left internal mammary artery, and thus may underestimate the long-term benefits of bypass surgery. They did reveal, though, that certain subgroups of patients live longer when they undergo bypass surgery. These patients can be categorized on an anatomical basis and include those with left main artery blockage; blockage of all three vessels when the heart muscle is weakened; and blockage of the origins of two vessels when one of them is the left anterior descending artery. Because of this improved longevity, whenever I have a patient possessing one of these anatomies, I usually recommend bypass surgery.

Bypass surgery is also extremely effective at decreasing the frequency of angina. In those patients who do not obtain symptomatic relief from either medications or angioplasty, bypass is a reasonable alternative. It can clearly improve a patient's lifestyle. We must remember that not all surgery is performed simply to prolong life. In fact, *most* surgeries like hernias, cataracts, and back surgery, are performed solely to improve lifestyle. Thus, when evaluating the appropriateness of bypass surgery, mortality is really not the only issue. Again, we must also consider lifestyle—the nature and frequency of the pain felt, what limits that pain places on a life, and how psychologically devastating recurrent angina can be. Happily, serious complications from bypass surgery are rare, occurring in only 1–3 percent of patients. They include infection, heart attack, stroke, and death.

Unfortunately, the only studies to compare mortality rates in angioplasty and bypass surgery came before the development of stents. In these studies, there was no appreciable difference in mortality between angioplasty and bypass patients. Perhaps now, with safer and more complete procedures providing lower restenosis rates, angioplasty might fare better than bypass surgery in patients with multivessel problems, but new comparison studies have yet to be done.

After bypass surgery, a large percentage of patients (75 percent in some studies) develop a transient decrease in thinking capacity, along with transient, mild visual deficits. It is interesting to note that although 90 percent of all patients achieve significant relief of their angina, many fewer patients actually return to prior employment. Does this suggest some relationship between work stress and the need for bypass surgery? Have these patients finally come to understand their own susceptibilities to work stress and the need to respond by altering their employment?

Bypass grafting in women merits special attention. In fact, debate has arisen over whether or not women are at greater risk during surgery solely because of gender. It now appears that this may be the case. Several studies have shown increased mortality and morbidity in women undergoing bypass surgery. Of course, women also tend to be sicker than men at the time of surgery. More specifically, statistics bear out a small increase in early postoperative deaths in women. Fortunately, late survival for both men and women is just about equivalent.

Nonetheless, with women experiencing less relief of anginal symptoms from bypass surgery, they do seem to achieve somewhat less benefit from it than men. Such considerations should not prevent a woman from undergoing coronary bypass grafting. Just as it is with men, bypass surgery can save a woman's life.

I'm sure you remember Mr. Goldberg from Chapter 1. Not "fitting" comfortably into any one of the three categories of angina treatment—drugs, angioplasty, or bypass—he was a perfect candidate for a natural approach to his disease. Had the "natural" or "integrative" additions we made to his usual regimen not relieved his angina, he might have needed a bypass strictly for relief of symptoms. But he fared well, had complete resolution of his symptoms, and so was able to avoid any further invasive, painful, or risky procedures.

In contrast, the case history of another patient, 65-year-old Jack Strom, illustrates just how valuable a bypass can be.

I received a call at midnight that Mr. Strom, a recently retired accountant, had flown from New York to Florida to be under the care of his own internist for the treatment of chest pain. Prior to leaving for New York, a doctor had given him nitroglycerine tablets to treat his newly developed chest pain. In the course of two days, while visiting relatives there, he'd taken nearly 100 nitroglycerine tablets!

I found him in the Emergency Room, ghostly pale, lying on a stretcher with his feet higher than his head because his blood pressure was a mere 70/40. Mr. Strom was dying. His EKG demonstrated diffuse ischemia—a huge area of his heart was being deprived of adequate blood flow. There was only one thing to do. I took him directly to the cardiac catheterization lab. What I discovered was astonishing: His left main coronary artery was totally blocked, and his left anterior descending and circumflex coronary arteries were being fed by nature's own bypasses—collateral blood flow—through the right coronary artery. Even worse, his right coronary artery—the only one still functioning at all—had a 95 percent blockage. I quickly inserted an intra-aortic balloon pump (IABP), a temporary device used to help improve the heart muscle's function in the setting of a dramatic and life-threatening cardiovascular event. Mr. Strom was rushed to the operating room, where he underwent multivessel coronary artery bypass grafting. Seven days later, he walked out of the hospital smiling, with a blood pressure of 130/70.

No herb, vitamin, mineral, or even pharmaceutical agent could have saved this man's life. The only intervention which could have, and did, was a bypass operation. Without the surgery, his wife would have been a widow and his children fatherless. When I attend alternative medicine conferences and hear people talk about abandoning bypass surgery, Mr. Strom and other patients like him come to mind. The heart surgeons are not our enemies, I tell these doctors, they are our friends. We must embrace them and hope they embrace alternative practitioners—as I have—to help find a common ground on which we may all work for the same goal: to improve our patients' lives.

On an experimental note, gene therapy and peripheral TMR (transmyocardial revascularization) possess some great possibilities. VEG-F, vascular endothelial growth factor (a product of genetic research), can be injected directly into the heart to help alleviate angina by stimulating the growth of new cardiac arteries. TMR employs a new laser to burn tiny holes through the heart muscle, developing new channels for blood vessel growth. This too can dramatically decrease angina. Let's keep our fingers crossed and hope that these and other procedures will result in clinically verifiable benefits for the many thousands of Americans inadequately treated by conventional methods.

Unstable Angina

Unstable angina bears several other, more revealing names. "Intermediate coronary syndrome" implies that this disorder lies between chronic stable angina and a heart attack (acute myocardial infarction). "Pre-infarction angina" is somewhat more ominous, implying the impending onset of a heart attack. "Crescendo angina" also carries forbidding implications. Strictly speaking, unstable angina is defined as the presence of one or more of the following (in the absence of an acute myocardial infarction):

1. A pattern of angina which is rapidly progressive, in that the frequency, severity, or duration of symptoms increases at an accelerating rate. This pattern is superimposed on a prior stable, chronic anginal pattern.
2. The presence of new-onset angina; that is, angina that never previously existed.
3. The presence of angina at rest; that is, angina in the absence of any significant physical activity.

The three symptoms of unstable angina signify a totally different physiology from that of chronic stable angina. In chronic stable angina, patients' symptoms occur when their hearts require an increasing amount of blood supply—when they exercise or during intense emotional stress. In the unstable angina patient, the problem is not one of an increase in demand, but rather a decrease in supply of blood to the heart. The arteries of an unstable angina patient have experienced an abrupt event, such as the rupture of a previously solid plaque, or the formation of a clot on top of a prior plaque. Vasospasm, or squeezing of a blood vessel, can also result in unstable angina.

These three events, which represent a decrease in the blood supply to the heart, leave the heart muscle starved for oxygen, culminating in the pain of angina pectoris.

Unstable angina is an enormous problem in the United States, with hundreds of thousands of patients admitted yearly to hospitals because of it. When assessing the coronary anatomy of these patients, it becomes apparent that they represent a typically "sick" population. In about 40 percent of these patients, all three vessels have significant blockages; in 20 percent two vessels possess significant blockage, and in 20 percent the left main artery—the most important vessel that feeds the heart—has a tight, life-threatening stenosis. Only 10 percent have but a single vessel involved, and another 10 percent have no lesion whatsoever. This latter population represents the 10 percent of the patients with unstable angina who have been misdiagnosed.

The natural history of unstable angina patients is not very promising. Almost 60 percent of these patients develop an "event" within eight months following their first symptoms. Patients who are older, have continued pain at rest, evidence of multivessel disease on angiography, or evidence of blood clots on angiography possess a particularly poor prognosis. If patients "cool down," however, and are able to undergo stress testing with normal results, we know that their risk is lower.

Currently, most all cardiologists treat unstable angina patients similarly. Depending on how sick they seem, patients are admitted to the hospital's coronary care or a slightly less intensive unit. They are placed on monitors to check their heart rhythms. To determine whether or not the patient has had a heart attack, blood tests and serial EKGs are done. Blood-thinning drugs, the mainstay of therapy, are used in tandem with nitrates and beta blockers, especially to reduce sudden episodes of angina. The common aspirin, which decreases platelet stickiness, can also reduce heart attacks and death by nearly 50 percent for such patients. Heparin, an intravenous form of blood thinner, decreases mortality and anginal episodes here as well, and is best used in conjunction with aspirin. For their part, the powerful blood thinning agent, thrombolytics, used effectively for heart attacks, does not benefit unstable angina patients.

TABLE 10
Medications Used to Treat Unstable Angina

Drug	Action	Potential Side Effects
Aspirin	Reduces heart attacks and death by nearly 50% in unstable angina patients.	• Thins the blood so that bleeding may occur. • Can irritate the lining of the gastrointestinal system.
Ticlid and Plavix	Like aspirin, these drugs decrease platelet stickiness (preventing blood clots), and may diminish heart attack deaths by nearly 50% in unstable angina patients.	• Thins the blood so that bleeding may occur. • Rarely, platelets may fall and "paradoxical blood clotting may occur.
Heparin	A "blood thinner" that decreases mortality and episodes of angina in unstable angina patients, especially when used with aspirin.	• Thins the blood so that bleeding may occur. • Rarely, platelets may fall and "paradoxical" blood clotting may occur.

After observing their patients for two or three days, most physicians encourage them to undergo cardiac catheterization so as to define their areas of blockage and the best treatment strategy.

After angiography, options include medical management, angioplasty (or other interventional techniques), and coronary artery bypass grafting. Not every patient is offered a choice. Certainly, the patient's coronary anatomy will help determine what his or her physician advises. With angioplasty, it is often beneficial to wait four to seven days while the patient remains on heparin, so as to diminish any possible risk to these patients. The only downside to this approach is an increase in hospital costs. At present, most hospitals discourage physicians from promoting this four- to seven-day extension. Additionally, studies have demonstrated improved results in unstable angina patients who undergo angioplasty when antiplatelet agents called glycoprotein IIB/IIIA platelet inhibitors are used. Reopro, which we discussed previously, is one such agent.

For patients who have undergone successful angioplasty in the treatment of unstable angina, long-term follow-up is very promising. In fact, the incidence of subsequent heart attacks drops as low as that of patients with chronic stable angina pectoris.

When patients are extremely ill and their anatomy does not permit angioplasty, they are often advised to undergo coronary artery bypass grafting. Unfortunately, because these patients are sicker than "stable" patients, the mortality of this procedure jumps to about 4 percent.

Even with this increase in mortality, studies show that the sickest patients, especially those who have "crossed over" from medical regimens to actual bypass surgery, benefit most from the surgery itself.

Now what of natural therapies in the management of unstable angina pectoris: Here is a case study that altered my perception of the strength of natural therapies as I hope it does yours.

Leonard Walsh was a previously healthy gentleman who developed unstable angina shortly after his seventy-seventh birthday. Needless to say, Mr. Walsh was admitted to the hospital in order to monitor his heart condition closely. As he continued to experience chest pain even after being given a variety of pharmaceutical agents, he was taken to the cardiac catheterization laboratory for a diagnostic angiogram. The test demonstrated a 90 percent blockage in his most important coronary artery. Extremely concerned that Mr.

Walsh would soon experience a substantial heart attack, I decided (with his approval) to implant a stent in his ailing artery. The procedure went well, and the blockage was reduced from 90 percent to approximately zero. Both he and I felt great.

Unfortunately, as is true with approximately 20 percent of all stent patients, Mr. Walsh returned six months later with a recurrent episode of chest discomfort, after having felt fine during the preceding period. A repeat angiogram proved what we had feared: His blockage had returned and, in fact, looked worse than it had prior to the stent. At this point, he and I decided to take a more natural approach. I placed him on a multivitamin, multimineral supplement with a high dose of antioxidant vitamins C and E, and a variety of other heart health-promoting antioxidants such as alpha lipoic acid, grape seed extract, and coenzyme Q-10. Important minerals for maintaining a healthy heart—such as magnesium, selenium, chromium, and copper—were also given at appropriate levels, as was the very important cardiac nutrient L-carnitine. I tried to convince Mr. Walsh to take a cholesterol-lowering pharmaceutical agent, but he was reluctant to "poison" his body with any medicine.

Mr. Walsh did very well until almost a year later, when he developed a different sort of chest discomfort. Although his symptoms had changed, I was so sure that his coronary artery disease had progressed that I took him directly to the cardiac catheterization laboratory. What we found shocked us. His previous, 90 percent, "awful-looking" blockage had been cleared to a mild 20–30 percent constriction. Never before had I ever witnessed such a dramatic regression of a coronary blockage. In fact, I was so astonished by his improvement that I showed Mr. Walsh's films to other invasive cardiologists. When asked how I had been able to improve Leonard's badly diseased vessel, my response was simply "vitamins." Although I cannot claim with certainty that the supplements he took cured his blockage, I can say that his artery dramatically improved, and that the only consistent change in his regimen was the addition of high-potency multivitamins and minerals. Perhaps the addition of powerful antioxidants and minerals allowed the body's inherent healing mechanisms to take over, effectively counteracting the tendency to form a blockage. Whatever the reason, his artery did demonstrate a dramatic recovery. Having observed the dramatic regression of his coronary disease, Mr.

Walsh is now filled with gratitude and confidence, and has become a devotee of natural medicine.

If Mr. Walsh's unstable angina had not been brought under control, he might have ended up at our final destination on the journey through coronary artery disease, the most serious of all—the acute myocardial infarction, a heart attack.

CHAPTER 6

Call 911—It's "The Big One"

Although death from heart attacks has decreased since 1960, myocardial infarction still remains a major health hazard, with over 1.5 million new heart attacks occurring annually in the United States—or one attack every twenty seconds! Of those patients who die from myocardial infarctions, usually the result of a lethal disturbance in heart rhythm, 50 percent pass away within the first hour of symptoms.

Since the 1960s though, several major developments have contributed to improvements here. First there was the creation of the modern coronary care unit, in which nurses monitor patients' heart rhythms, ensuring prompt responses to potentially lethal rhythms. We also now know that with aspirin and beta blockers we can reduce the risks of heart attacks. Thrombolytics, powerful agents given intravenously to break up the culprit clot causing a heart attack, can also diminish mortality. Angioplasty, previously considered too dangerous to perform during a heart attack, is now the best method of treatment.

Unfortunately, even with such beneficial tools, the three most effective—thrombolytics, aspirin, and beta blockers—are still underutilized by too many physicians in America. Calcium channel blockers, on the other hand, which in comparison are not as effective for acute myocardial infarction, are overutilized also by too many physicians.

Early treatment is the key here, especially in managing an acute myocardial infarction. As a medical resident at Bellevue Hospital in New York City, I well recall our motto when dealing with heart attack victims: "time is muscle." We often competed, desperately trying to be the quickest team to start thrombolytic therapy in our heart attack patients. As I stated earlier, most deaths from heart attacks occur within the first hour after developing symptoms. Unfortunately, many of those who die do so needlessly. If they had simply recognized their symptoms as being potentially life-threatening, they would have immeasurably increased their chance of surviving. Delays in diagnosis generally occur because patients hesitate before seeking help.

What factors predispose to the delayed diagnosis of a heart attack? A number of factors appear again and again: (1) old age, (2) diabetes, (3) mild symptoms, (4) nighttime heart attacks, (5) living alone, and (6) involvement of a general practitioner prior to going to an emergency room. Again, some treatments work only when administered immediately; for example, the greatest benefit from thrombolytic therapy occurs within the first 60–90 minutes after symptoms begin. Thus, it is paramount that patients learn to recognize the symptoms of a heart attack. Your life may depend on how appropriate and prompt your treatment is.

The Causes of Heart Attacks

What causes this devastating cardiovascular event? Atherosclerosis, or plaque formation, allows for an active blockage to build up in an artery, which then leads to the development of a heart attack. In nearly all heart attack victims, the common denominator is the presence of a blood clot inside a blood vessel.

The clot (thrombus) generally forms on top of a preexisting plaque that has ruptured, exposing substances inside the plaque to blood vessel elements. Since the blood products and plaque components don't "mix," blood clots develop.

"Nonatherosclerotic" heart attacks occur only rarely, but they are not unheard of. Some of the more interesting causes of these "non-plaque" heart attacks include cocaine and oral contraceptive use, syphilis involving the aorta, and complications of a cardiac catheterization (angiogram). These nonatherosclerotic heart attacks represent, at most, 6 percent of all heart attacks.

Diagnosis and Treatment of Heart Attacks

To diagnose a myocardial infarction, physicians must demonstrate two of the three following findings:

1. The patient must have the classic symptom complex of a heart attack which includes a pain like that of angina pectoris which is unremitting and lasts longer than thirty minutes.
2. Typical EKG changes must be observed.
3. Blood enzymes which can be released from damaged heart muscle must be found to be elevated, and then return to their baseline levels.

As a heart attack means *death* of heart muscle, this is a time of urgency for both the physician and the patient. When a patient is having a heart attack, our goal is to limit the degree of damage inflicted on the heart. The less damage, the better the patient's prognosis will be.

Of course, to receive the greatest benefit, patients must be treated efficiently and immediately. Once they hit the emergency room, a lightning-fast triage must occur, enabling the medical team to determine how sick the patient is and what treatment to follow (see Tables 11 and 12). Patients are placed on cardiac monitors, oxygen administered, and medications given, including aspirin, heparin, nitroglycerine, and beta blockers. Pain medicines are also critical, as they help to limit levels of circulating blood hormones like epinephrine and norepinephrine that could otherwise potentially stimulate lethal heart rhythms during an attack. Avoid calcium channel blockers; they present potential problems for heart attack patients.

Diagnostic Signs of a Heart Attack:
What You and Your Doctor Should Look For

- The symptoms of angina pectoris ("squeezing" pressure in the chest, tightness or pain radiating from the chest to the neck, jaw, or either arm, along with any of the syndrome's unusual symptoms) unremittingly for more than thirty minutes.
- Changes in the patient's EKG that signal a heart attack has occurred.
- Changes in the patient's blood enzymes that show the heart muscle has been damaged.

As potent blood thinners, thrombolytics have become the main-stay of therapy for the heart attack victim. These agents were first uti-lized on an intracoronary basis—in other words, they were directly administered, via catheters, into the blocked arteries feeding the heart. Currently, they are administered through regular IVs (in a vein in the arm, for example). By improving heart muscle function, thrombolytics have clearly improved survival in heart attack patients. Unfortunately, there may be complications, including bleeding. Pa-tients over the age of 65, or those with significantly elevated blood pressure, also have an increased risk of bleeding into their brains (intracranial bleeding). This complication can be devastating, lead-ing to permanent brain damage or even death. Overall, however, even with that potential complication, thrombolytic drugs signifi-cantly improve mortality statistics in heart attack victims.

I must reiterate that early treatment with thrombolytic therapy is much more effective than late treatment. In fact, several studies have demonstrated the *absence* of any life-saving benefit in the late use of thrombolytics. Such drugs must be taken within the first 6–12 hours after the onset of symptoms.

Another extremely effective approach in treating heart attacks in-volves the use of primary angioplasty—that is, using angioplasty as a first treatment. In these patients, there's a lower risk of intracranial bleeding and blood vessels regain more of their functionality com-pared to patients treated with thrombolytic agents. Additionally, re-search has shown a 40 percent drop in short-term mortality when comparing angioplasty to thrombolytic therapy.

Reading this, you must be thinking that angioplasty is clearly the better approach, and so it is. Yet fewer than 20 percent of the hospi-tals in America have the capability of performing primary angio-plasty. Thus, although primary angioplasty is likely the better treatment option for heart attack patients, the majority of patients are sadly out of luck here.

A "back to the future" treatment for heart attack, first tested in the 1960s then discarded, may be making a comeback. This treatment is a combination of glucose, insulin, and potassium. The theory is that giving a heart attack victim insulin draws glucose and energy into the heart. Potassium is part of the regimen because, anytime a person takes insulin, potassium (like glucose) is pulled into their cells, so circulating potassium is depleted. Recently, this regimen was tested on 407 people having heart attacks. The death rate in the treated group was decreased significantly compared to heart attack victims who weren't treated with this combination of substances. In hospitals where primary angioplasty isn't available, the glucose, insulin, and potassium regimen could be an excellent—and relatively inexpensive—alternative.

Once the heart attack patient has been started on thrombolytic therapy or has undergone primary angioplasty, he or she is transferred to the coronary care unit (CCU). The CCU embodies one of the greatest advances in modern medicine's treatment of acute coronary artery syndromes. The nursing care administered to these high-risk patients has truly been life-saving. It is not just the observation of

TABLE 11
Primary Treatment of Acute Myocardial Infarction (Heart Attack)

Drug/Procedure Used	Action
Cardiac monitor	Monitors the beating of the heart and alerts doctors and nurses when it becomes irregular.
Oxygen	Helps the patient breathe easily, and allows the heart not to work as hard.
Pain medication	Helps control the pain from the heart attack, as well as diminishing the amount of circulating stress hormones (epinephrine and norepinephrine) that can cause the heart to beat erratically.
Thrombolytic drugs	Administered through an IV, these drugs break up the blood clots that precipitate most heart attacks. To be most effective, they must be administered within 6–12 hours after the onset of the heart attack. Treatment with thrombolytics has clearly improved survival from heart attacks. In people over the age of 65, there is an increased possibility of these drugs causing bleeding into the brain; angioplasty is another option for individuals at risk of this complication.
Angioplasty	Primary angioplasty—using this procedure as the first treatment for heart attacks—diminishes the possible complication of bleeding in the brain, and results in a 40% drop in short-term mortality. However, fewer than 20% of American hospitals are equiped to perform primary angioplasty.

TABLE 12
Secondary Treatment of Acute Myocardial Infarction (Heart Attack)

Drug/Procedure Used	Action
Beta blockers (Tenormin, Lopressor)	Definitely decrease mortality when used at the time of an acute heart attack.
Angiotensin converting enzyme inhibitors ("ACE inhibitors," like Vasotec, Captopril, Zestril)	Decrease mortality in both high- and low-risk patients when used at the time of an acute heart attack. Even more effective when added to a regimen consisting of aspirin and a beta blocker.
Aspirin	Decreases platelet stickiness, thereby decreasing the risk of another heart attack.
Nitrates (nitroglycerine)	Allow the heart to use oxygen more efficiently, and make platelets less sticky, reducing the risk of another heart attack.

patients' rhythm disturbances, or the careful monitoring of blood pressure and heart rate, that has made this unit so very valuable. The actual "laying on" of hands has also been demonstrated to be beneficial for patients. For example, studies have shown that when CCU nurses have gently and confidently "laid hands" upon heart attack patients, sympathetic tone has been diminished (epinephrine and norepinephrine levels have been decreased) and, therefore, blood pressure and heart rate elevation and rhythm disturbances have also occurred less frequently.

Lowering Mortality from Heart Attacks After They Occur

- Early diagnosis and treatment
- Use of thrombolytic drugs to break up clots in blood vessels
- Angioplasty
- Beta blockers
- ACE inhibitors
- Magnesium

Many pharmacologic agents other than thrombolytics have been studied in treating acute myocardial infarctions, and some have actually been shown to possess mortality-reducing benefits. Beta blockers are the oldest and probably the best analyzed of all these drugs. In a review of over 27 studies, including over 27,000 patients, mortality was found to decrease in those patients treated with beta blockers at the time of their heart attack.

Researchers have also found angiotensin converting enzyme inhibitors (ACE inhibitors) to decrease death from acute myocardial infarctions. In a review of eight mortality trials evaluating ACE inhibitors in treating acute myocardial infarctions, researchers found reductions in the incidence of death in both high- and low-risk patients. Researchers also demonstrated that the addition of an ACE inhibitor to a preexisting regimen of beta blockers and aspirin resulted in an even greater improvement in mortality than with just beta blockers and aspirin. Thus, I, for one, recommend that all patients with acute myocardial infarctions be treated with beta blockers, aspirin, and ACE inhibitors. In those patients with significant left ventricular dysfunction, ACE inhibitors should be continued for life. When minimal heart damage has occurred, ACE inhibitors can be discontinued several months after a heart attack.

Patients with an uncomplicated course and whose symptoms resolve without recurrence usually transfer from the CCU within one or two days into a telemetry unit—again for continuous monitoring of heart rates and rhythms. The patient who suffers from an uncomplicated heart attack may be discharged from the hospital within five to seven days of the onset of symptoms.

Complications of Heart Attacks

Since heart attacks are so common, and their effects so devastating, it's important to discuss a few of the more common and disastrous complications. Within the first day or two, early complications include a drop in blood pressure and altered heart rhythms. These can usually be addressed with the administration of fluids and medications respectively (see Table 13).

When a great deal of heart muscle has been jeopardized, patients can develop congestive heart failure, resulting in the accumulation of fluid in the lungs. Not only is this experience extremely uncomfortable, but it can be life-threatening. It is generally treated with medications, including diuretics and other pharmacologic agents, aimed at increasing the inotropy (strength of contractility) of the heart muscle.

A rare group of patients develops the extreme version of congestive heart failure, called "cardiogenic shock." In these patients, blood pressure falls precipitously and the lungs flood with fluid. Most of these individuals have severe, three-vessel coronary disease, and the majority of them die from their heart attacks with or without aggressive therapy.

A more common untoward cardiovascular event involves the rupture of various portions of the heart, which is the consequence of tissue death. At times, the free wall of the heart can tear, sending blood into the pericardial space that lines the heart, resulting in death 90 percent of the time. At other times, the wall of the heart that separates the two ventricles (the ventricular septum) can rupture, a condition called a "ventricular septal defect" (VSD). This, too, usually follows three to six days after a heart attack, resulting in death 90 percent of the time. Fortunately, when these patients can be transferred to a hospital with the capacity for appropriate surgical intervention, the death rate can be decreased to as low as 50 percent.

In papillary muscle rupture, a portion of a muscle which holds part of the mitral valve in place will tear. As with a VSD (ventricular septal defect), there is a 90 percent mortality without surgery and approximately a 50 percent mortality with surgery. Fortunately, all three of these dramatic devastations of heart muscle are rare.

Rhythm disturbances can also occur in a small group of heart attack victims. Depending upon the rhythm abnormality, physicians have several therapeutic options available. At times, observation alone is sufficient. Otherwise, patients may require the transient use of pharmacologic agents or temporary and sometimes even permanent pacemakers.

An unusual complication of a heart attack, Dressler's syndrome, can occur within one to eight weeks afterward. Although it is not wholly clear what causes this problem, we do know this disorder is systemic, perhaps caused by the formation of antibodies to one's own heart. Dressler's syndrome symptoms include a feeling of weakness and malaise with possible fever and high white blood counts. Aspirin is the mainstay of therapy here. Fortunately, Dressler's syndrome is rare and usually short-lived.

When patients are unfortunate enough to have experienced an extremely large heart attack, clots can accumulate within the left ventricle, the main pumping chamber of the heart. The obvious concern here relates to the possibility of the blood clot's traveling from the left heart into a distant part of the body, like the brain, kidneys, or spleen. Echocardiographic assessment of these blood clots has enabled us to determine which ones are more likely to travel (embolize) than others. Current treatment involves Coumadin, an oral blood thinner, for at least three to six months after the attack when a clot is noted on an echocardiogram. Treatment can also involve aspirin, as well as Coumadin, to decrease the frequency of future cardiovascular events. Coumadin can usually be discontinued three to six months after the heart attack.

Fortunately, all of the above complications are relatively uncommon, and a typical heart attack victim will be able to leave the hospital within a week in a relatively unscathed condition. Prior to departing the hospital, patients should receive counseling about lifestyle changes such as stress modification and dietary adjustments. Several weeks after discharge, the patient usually undergoes a mild stress test to enroll him or her in a cardiac rehabilitation program. Cardiac rehabilitation is important not only for physical conditioning but also as a means of providing psychological support during what is often a very emotionally wrenching time.

TABLE 13
Potential Complications of Acute Myocardial Infarction (Heart Attack)

Complication	Treatment
Drop in blood pressure	• Blood pressure–elevating medications; fluids.
Heart rhythm abnormalities	• Drug therapy to restore the heart's steady rhythm.
Congestive heart failure (CHF)	• Diuretics, to remove excess fluid from the lungs and other areas where it can accumulate. • Drugs to increase the strength of the heart's contraction.
Cardiogenic shock (extreme congestive heart failure)	• May involve actual tearing of heart muscle or valve, which requires surgical repair. • Drugs as with CHF • IABP

Natural Methods of Treating Heart Attack Patients

The many benefits of medical technology are clear. Additionally, however, there are several, very helpful natural approaches that I have found for treating heart attacks. Here then is a story about the changing nature of medicine.

Nitrates, which we discussed previously, possess many benefits that may also aid a patient having an acute myocardial infarction. When using nitrates, myocardial oxygen requirements are less. In response, and as a side benefit of taking nitroglycerine, platelets become less sticky. Trials, in fact, have demonstrated a possibly small mortality benefit with the use of nitroglycerine during an acute myocardial infarction. During my residency in the mid-1980s, I recall the chief cardiologist at New York University chastising me for using nitroglycerine for a heart attack patient. He stated that there was no documented evidence for its use, and at the time he was right. Since then there have been numerous studies elucidating the potential benefits of nitrates in treating heart attacks, with nitrates now the standard of care.

I tell this story more to highlight the evolution of medicine than anything else. Medicine changes continuously, its rules being rewritten sometimes on a daily basis. Such understanding is essential, especially in regard to natural modalities for treating heart disease patients. Too many traditional doctors blindly dismiss the possible benefits of naturally based treatment strategies. Fortunately for us, there is already sufficient evidence to justify their use in many circumstances. There are also trials now ongoing that will continue to support their use; and personally, in my own practice, I have found many natural remedies to be extraordinarily effective at decreasing some complications of coronary artery disease and peripheral vascular disease. Again, ours is an ongoing journey during which we constantly must be learning, reassessing, and reevaluating our own basic tools and approaches to disease.

For example, the mineral magnesium has been evaluated in numerous studies of acute myocardial infarction patients. We know that heart attack victims tend to have low levels of magnesium, usually a result of lower dietary intake, advanced age, and the use of diuretics in this particular patient population. In fact, several larger studies have shown that three-quarters of the American population may actually be deficient in magnesium. Thus, we need not search for a unique causative factor to explain why heart attack patients are depleted of magnesium; it is enough that they live in America.

By 1990, over 1,500 patients had been randomized in trials which demonstrated a nearly 50 percent reduction in mortality when magnesium was administered *early on* in the setting of a heart attack. Unfortunately, ISIS 4, an extremely large study, demonstrated no significant improvement with the administration of magnesium. This study has been wrongly used by many opponents of "natural medicine" as a justification to abandon the use of magnesium in the treatment of a heart attack. They are in error. In ISIS 4, researchers gave the magnesium very late, on average twelve hours after the onset of a heart attack, making comparisons of this with previous trials quite impractical. On the other hand, we can say that heart attack victims given magnesium as late as twelve hours after onset may not receive much benefit.

I feel that, in the absence of any contraindications such as low blood pressure or kidney disease, magnesium should be administered to all heart attack patients. It is a benign agent and has a great potential benefit.

While recovering from a heart attack, lifestyle modifications are paramount (see Table 14). Patients must honestly evaluate their lives and adjust them to improve not only their overall life expectancy, but their enjoyment of life's pleasures. This includes developing ways to limit stress, whether it is through meditation, exercise, yoga, T'ai Chi, or aromatherapy.

TABLE 14
Lifestyle Modifications to Make After Having a Heart Attack

Lifestyle Change	How to Start
Limit stress	• Meditation. • Yoga. • T'ai Chi. • Aromatherapy. • Freeze frame.
Exercise	• 30–40 minutes of aerobic workout daily benefits physical and emotional condition. • Exercise methods like T'ai Chi can both decrease stress and improve fitness.

TABLE 14 (Continued)
Lifestyle Modifications to Make After Having a Heart Attack

Dietary adjustments	• Decrease saturated fat. • Increase vegetables and fruits. • Increase nuts and seeds. • Decrease trans-fats (such as margarine). • Increase omega-3 fatty acids by eating fatty fish (such as salmon). • Decrease intake of sugary foods.

Dietary adjustments are also fundamental. One must decrease the amount of saturated fat consumed and increase the intake of vegetables, fruits, nuts, and seeds. Exercise is also critical. A daily exercise regimen incorporating thirty to forty minutes of an aerobic workout will help all individuals, not just those who suffer from coronary disease. Exercise serves not simply to improve one's physical condition, but also to benefit one's emotional state.

Nutritional supplements can further afford a great benefit to those with risk factors for coronary disease, as well as those who already suffer from it (see Table 15). In later chapters, I will discuss the many benefits of these nutritional supplements. For now, I will simply mention several of my favorites. Vitamin E and vitamin C are potent fat-soluble and water-soluble antioxidants, respectively, which have been shown to limit the development of cardiovascular events. Gugul and garlic are herbs which have been found to be beneficial in lowering cholesterol. Betaine or trimethylglycine, in addition to vitamins B_6, B_{12}, and folic acid, decreases homocysteine levels, which will most likely translate into lessening the development of coronary disease. Hawthorn is an herb which has many cardiovascular benefits, such as lowering blood pressure, decreasing the stickiness of platelets, and improving the contractility of the heart muscle. Coenzyme Q-10 and L-carnitine are supplements which can improve energy creation and use by our hearts and skeletal muscles.

The omega-3 fatty acids, EPA and DHA, have been shown to lower triglycerides, lower blood pressure, and decrease the stickiness of our blood. These fatty acids have many other great benefits that we'll discuss in more detail later, including improving nerve function and painful joints in arthritic patients.

Psyllium, pectin, and guar gum are water-soluble fibers which can benefit not only our gastrointestinal tracts, but also our cholesterol profiles, by decreasing total cholesterol and LDL cholesterol. These fibers have also been shown to stabilize blood sugar levels in diabetics and to decrease blood pressure in hypertensive patients.

Finally, taurine and arginine are two amino acids which also have potential benefit for cardiovascular disease patients. Taurine has been shown to lower blood pressure in several studies and also has purportedly helped patients with various rhythm disturbances. On a personal basis, however, I have found magnesium to be more effective in treating rhythm disorders such as atrial fibrillation and benign PVCs. Arginine is a precursor of nitric oxide and thus at high doses will help arterial blood vessels release nitric oxide and improve their ability to dilate. This can benefit patients who suffer not only from coronary artery disease but also from congestive heart failure.

TABLE 15
Natural Remedies for Heart Attack Patients

Vitamin/Mineral	Action
Magnesium	Heart attack patients are low in magnesium; administering magnesium early in treatment of heart attacks can produce as much as a 50% decrease in mortality. Administering magnesium later in treatment may not produce as great a benefit, but is still helpful to the patient. Magnesium relaxes blood vessels and lowers blood pressure.
Vitamin E	A potent fat-soluble antioxidant vitamin that helps limit development of cardiac disease.
Vitamin C	A potent water-soluble antioxidant that contributes to heart health.
Gugul	An herb that helps lower cholesterol.
Garlic	An herb that helps to lower cholesterol levels and blood pressure.

TABLE 15 (Continued)
Natural Remedies for Heart Attack Patients

Vitamin/Mineral	Action
B vitamins: B_6, B_{12}, and folic acid	Help to lower homocysteine levels; high homocysteine is now recognized as an important risk factor for developing heart disease.
Water-soluble fiber: psyllium, pectin, and guar gum	Benefits gastrointestinal tract, and helps decrease both total and LDL cholesterol. This type of fiber also stabilizes blood sugar levels in diabetics and decreases high blood pressure.
Hawthorn	This herb lowers blood pressure, decreases stickiness of platelets, and helps the heart muscle work more efficiently.
Carnitine	Helps the heart use energy more efficiently.
Coenzyme Q-10	Helps the heart use energy more efficiently.
Omega-3 fatty acids (EPA and DHA)	Decrease blood platelet stickiness, lower triglycerides, and lower blood pressure. These fatty acids also improve arthritis symptoms.
Amino acids: taurine and arginine	Help to lower blood pressure and contribute to heart health.

A quick comment on chelation therapy: An alternative approach in the management of atherosclerotic disease (both coronary and peripheral), chelation therapy utilizes intravenous EDTA as a means of removing "free" metal ions from the body. Excess iron, copper, and calcium are scavenged in an attempt to limit their free-radical damaging effects on our arteries. Although this process sounds promising, there is a dearth of data supporting its benefits. When performed properly, however, this is at least a safe process. As there are many anecdotal reports of its great efficacy, and in view of its safety, I usually advise my "medical" coronary patients who are interested in this procedure that, if they desire to undergo chelation, it must be performed by a doctor trained by the American College of Advancement of Medicine (ACAM). Although I do not practice chelation, I believe it may possess some benefit, particularly in light of its widespread use (over 500,000 people have been chelated in the last twenty to thirty years), and its popular support among countless patients and doctors. I must emphatically state, however, that I do *not* consider chelation a replacement for bypass surgery or angioplasty. When a clearly established traditional therapy has been proved to provide life-saving benefits, I believe it should be utilized as a "first" option, not a choice of last resort. Chelation can be reserved for those patients who are either to be medically managed, or who are poor candidates for more accepted and documented procedures. Hopefully, future studies will clarify chelation's role in the management of coronary artery disease.

CHAPTER 7

Heart Failure: When the Muscle Doesn't Squeeze

The heart is a pump, and its power lies within the muscle. Unfortunately, there are many ways in which the heart muscle can fail, producing a condition called "congestive heart failure." Currently, 2 million Americans receive treatment for congestive heart failure, and every year an additional 400,000 Americans develop it. What does it mean to have a failing heart—to be in congestive heart failure?

First off, heart failure is not synonymous with a heart attack; in fact, they are completely different. Congestive heart failure occurs when the heart is unable to keep up with the demands placed on it. In other words, the failing heart cannot pump enough blood forward. As some of the blood "backs up," fluid accumulates, flooding various regions of the body. The lack of sufficient blood flow to various tissues can result in symptoms such as difficulty in breathing or thinking and kidney failure.

What Happens in Heart Failure?

For your own ease in understanding, let's refer to the diagram of the heart that we used in Chapter 2.

Focus on the left ventricle, the chamber of the heart most likely to fail. If the left ventricle functions inadequately, arterial blood (the blood that should be pumped "forward" to nourish the rest of the body) will back up into the left atrium, the pulmonary arteries, and subsequently, the lungs. As the heart continues to fail, blood pres-

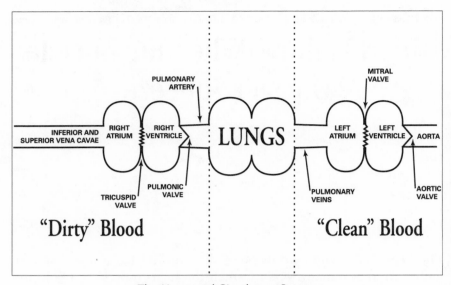

The Heart and Circulatory System

sure increases within the lungs, and fluid can accumulate in the air spaces that should contain *only* air. This "pulmonary edema" is extraordinarily uncomfortable. Patients feel as if they are drowning in their own fluids.

As an extreme version of congestive heart failure, pulmonary edema is often viewed as "backward" failure, in which blood backs up and collects because of the left ventricle's inability to push it "forward." Backward failure does not usually exist in isolation, but in combination with "forward failure."

The concept of *forward* failure implies that the heart muscle is failing to pump blood effectively, resulting in inadequate delivery of blood to the tissues. We know that the entire body—brain, liver, spleen, kidneys, and skeletal muscles—is dependent upon the heart's ability to pump blood effectively. As the heart's capacity to pump is hindered, forward failure results. When various tissues receive an inadequate supply of nourishing arterial blood, a spectrum of symptoms and disorders can result. For instance, an inadequate delivery of blood to the brain can cause fatigue and sluggish mental processes. When blood flow to the kidneys is limited, kidney failure occurs; and when blood flow to the skeletal muscles is reduced, weakness and easy fatigability ensue.

Thus far, we have been discussing failure of the *left* ventricle, which causes "left heart failure." What happens when the *right* ventricle fails? The outcome is—you guessed it—"right heart failure."

In *backward right heart failure* venous blood begins to pool throughout the body. Patients develop extreme swelling of their legs, fluid within their bellies (i.e., the peritoneum), and oftentimes swollen and painful livers.

Forward right heart failure causes an inadequate delivery of blood to the lungs and subsequently to the left heart, resulting in symptoms similar to those of forward left heart failure.

As our left and right ventricles are connected and work very much as a team, it is commoner to have combined left and right heart failure than it is to have left or right heart failure alone. There are, of course, circumstances when isolated right or left heart failure will occur, but they are well beyond the scope of our discussion.

In congestive heart failure, it is necessary to understand the distinction between systolic and diastolic dysfunction. You may recall from Chapter 2 that "systole" is the period during which the ventricles contract, whereas "diastole" is the time when the ventricles relax. Systolic heart failure refers to the heart's inability to squeeze adequately; diastolic dysfunction refers to the heart's inability to relax.

In diastolic dysfunction, the heart is stiff (i.e., unrelaxed) and thus unable to *accept* enough blood, resulting in significant backward failure. It turns out that about one-third of all patients with heart failure have pure diastolic dysfunction, one-third have pure systolic dysfunction, and one-third experience combined systolic and diastolic dysfunction. Thus heart failure does not necessarily imply a "weak" heart muscle. Often, it is simply an inability of the heart to *relax* that leads to congestive heart failure.

The Body's Response to Heart Failure

When a patient's heart begins to fail, his body attempts to protect itself. In the short run, these responses are beneficial but in the long run, they can be devastating, leading to a vicious cycle that ultimately results in worsening heart failure and even death.

What are these "short-sighted" responses? First and foremost, via the sympathetic nervous system, is the stress-activated "fight or flight" response. As a precise response to the the heart's ineffectiveness, the body seeks to retain its fluids and tightens the blood vessels (or vasoconstricts) as it does so. At the same time, blood is shunted to the brain and the heart at the expense of the kidneys, skin, and large skeletal muscles, etc. Although decreased blood flow to skeletal muscles leads to weakness and fatigue, preferential flow to the heart and brain allows these vital organs to continue functioning.

By responding to this stress, the body decreases its capacity to relax, which can also lead to a lowering of heart rate variability—a condition often associated with sudden cardiac death. It is also interesting to note that while blood levels of norepinephrine increase two- to threefold over normal levels (because of the increase in the "fight or flight" response), local heart levels are actually reduced, perhaps weakening the heart further.

During this time, there is also a decrease or "down regulation" of cardiac beta receptors. The discovery of this "down-regulation" was just what researchers needed to show that beta-blocker drugs might actually help patients who suffer from heart failure. (We'll discuss this unexpected phenomenon later in the chapter.)

The thickening (hypertrophy) of the heart muscle and dilatation of the ventricle (an increase in the chamber size) comprise the two, final automatic mechanisms that cause short-term improvement in heart failure patients.

When the heart muscle hypertrophies, or increases in size, it does not add new cells, but instead enlarges preexisting cells. The mitochondria (the powerhouses of the cells) have the awesome responsibility of providing energy to the heart muscle cells. When hearts enlarge, mitochondria also increase significantly in size, but not in number. There is one fascinating theory of heart failure that focuses upon this fact: As the heart increases in size—and concomitantly, in energy requirement—there comes a point at which the mitochondria can no longer keep up with its increased demands and crash all at once—resulting in more extreme heart failure.

The mitochondrial theory of heart failure also helps explain why certain natural substances such as coenzyme Q-10 and L-carnitine (both essential in proper mitochondrial function) are so helpful in treating and managing heart failure patients. Both of these naturally occurring substances are essential for proper functioning of our bodies' ubiquitous energy-producing units, the mitochondria. By augmenting our hearts' levels of these substances, the enhanced production of energy can cause weakened hearts to function at higher levels.

We must also not forget nature's other gifts that can aid in the treatment of heart failure (see Table 16). For example, magnesium, our body's natural calcium channel blocker, not only dilates blood vessels, but also helps our hearts function more efficiently. Hawthorn, an herb with remarkable cardiovascular benefits (described in greater detail in Chapter 13), both eases the burden on our hearts and dilates (or expands) our blood vessels, leading to overall improvement in heart muscle function. L-arginine, an amino acid, is the precursor to nitric oxide, a naturally occurring vasodilator normally produced by our coronary arteries. Supplementing with L-arginine can increase levels of nitric oxide, resulting in improved heart muscle function and diminished symptoms of heart failure. Thiamin (vitamin B_1) has clearly been demonstrated to improve heart muscle function in those patients deficient in this essential nutrient.

TABLE 16
Natural Remedies That Can Help Manage Congestive Heart Failure

Natural Supplements	Recommended Daily Dosage
L-carnitine	1–2 g twice daily
Coenzyme Q-10	200 to 400 mg daily in two divided doses
Magnesium	400 mg daily
Thiamin	100 mg daily
Hawthorn extract	160–900 mg of leaf, flower extract
L-arginine	2–4 g three times daily on an empty stomach
Omega-3 fatty acids	3 g daily of EPA and DHA (combined)

The Heart Muscle Diseases (Cardiomyopathies)

Unfortunately, over recent years the frequency of cardiomy-opathies has increased significantly in the United States. Although there are 3 major categories of cardiomyopathies, only 2 are common enough to describe in this chapter. In its most common form, or dilated cardiomyopathy (DCM), the heart enlarges, weakens, and grows flabby. An insidious disease that can go untreated for some time, DCM usually culminates in severe congestive heart failure.

Hypertrophic cardiomyopathies (HCM) refer to another group of diseases in which the heart muscle thickens while sustaining or even increasing its capacity to squeeze (intropy).

In the third and rarest form, restrictive cardiomyopathy (RCM), the dysfunction rests in the heart's inability to fill appropriately (i.e., diastolic dysfunction). Causes of RCM can include infiltrative muscle diseases such as scleroderma, sarcoid, amyloid, and metastatic cancer. We will begin our exploration of cardiomyopthy with its most common form: dilated cardiomyopathy.

Dilated Cardiomyopathy

Idiopathic dilated cardiomyopathy (IDCM) is far and away the commonest cause of the dilated cardiomyopathies. "Idiopathic" means that the cause of the condition is never clearly established. Currently there are 5–8 cases per 100,000 people per year, but again, this trend is rising. IDCM is much commoner in men in general and African-American men specifically. Survival is also significantly worse in African-Americans than in Caucasians, for unknown reasons.

The "natural history" of the disorder is also difficult to establish, because asymptomatic patients usually do not appear in a doctor's office. It is known, however, that once the disease is diagnosed, symptomatic patients fare much worse than asymptomatic patients. In fact, patients with symptoms of heart failure due to idiopathic dilated cardiomyopathy have a 25 percent chance of dying within one year, and a 50 percent chance of mortality in five years.

Although it is extremely difficult to predict which individual patients will fare well and which will not, there are several characteristics to watch out for. An increase in heart size, a decrease in heart muscle function, and the presence of symptoms definitely don't augur well. Patients with poor exercise capacity also have a particularly dismal prognosis. Of course, I am speaking generally here. If you have been told that you or a loved one suffers from any form of heart failure (or any type of heart disease), you should rely on your own doctor's assessment of your condition. Every patient is an individual, requiring individual diagnosis and treatment that cannot be gained from the pages of a book.

TABLE 17
Types of Heart Muscle Diseases (Cardiomyopathies)

Disease	What Goes Wrong
Dilated cardiomyopathy (DCM)	The heart enlarges, weakens, and grows flabby. It's unknown what causes the commonest form of this disease, which is why it's called "idiopathic dilated cardiomyopathy," or IDCM. Symptoms include inability to exercise, tiring easily, progressive weakness, and shortness of breath with exertion, progressing to severe debilitation. This condition can culminate in severe congestive heart failure.
Hypertrophic cardiomyopathy (HCM)	The heart muscle thickens, but continues to beat strongly. This disorder often has no symptoms, but when they occur, they can include shortness of breath, chest pain, fatigue, and lightheadedness. Most patients have nearly normal life expectancies.
Restrictive cardiomyopathy (RCM)	In this rare disease, the heart is unable to fill properly with blood, and so cannot pump blood to the rest of the body. It is very rarely seen in the Western hemisphere.

Although the cause of IDCM is usually unknown, three mechanisms are suspected of leading to its genesis:

1. Familial or genetic factors have been shown to be present in approximately 20 percent of all patients. A rare form of carnitine deficiency is one example of a genetic disorder leading to a cardiomyopathy. In this disease, patients with low carnitine levels (carnitine helps to transport fats across mitochondrial membranes) improve dramatically when given supplements. This is another ex-

ample of how taking an open-minded, "natural" approach to medicine—practicing integrative medicine, as I do—can result in finding a natural, nontoxic, noninvasive treatment for a potentially serious condition.

2. A viral etiology has been a longtime favorite of the academic world. It is known that undetected viral infections of the heart muscle (myocarditis) may, in fact, initiate an autoimmune response which subsequently attacks our hearts. Proponents of this theory point to the fact that high levels of antiviral antibodies have been found in some patients with IDCM. Opponents point out that other studies show most patients without infected myocardia. Additional studies show that when assessing patients with myocarditis, only 15 percent actually progress to dilated cardiomyopathy, making viral causation much less likely.

3. Abnormalities in immune function is a third mechanism thought to cause dilated cardiomyopathy. Such abnormalities have been documented in some patients with dilated cardiomyopathies, but is not yet considered a common cause of the disorder.

What fate awaits the typical patient with a dilated cardiomyopathy? The typical patient is a middle-aged male who comes to his doctor with minimal symptoms, such as a diminished exercise capacity, easy fatigability, progressive weakness, and shortness of breath on exertion. These symptoms may insidiously progress until the patient becomes severely debilitated. It is important to recognize that any patient who develops DCM should be evaluated for reversible causes such as low phosphate or calcium, or abnormal thyroid function. Cardiologists follow their patients' progress by using echocardiograms or radionuclide ventriculograms (nuclear scans looking at heart muscle function) every six to twelve months. We generally see patients with cardiomyopathies every three to four months to ensure their stability. I will discuss further management of the condition with medications later in this chapter.

A common, preventable, and "nonidiopathic" cause of heart muscle dysfunction is alcohol abuse. Alcohol, a particularly potent heart toxin, leads to 33 percent of all dilated cardiomyopathy cases in the United States. It is estimated that two-thirds of all American adults consume alcohol, and 10 percent of all adults consume heavy quantities of alcohol, creating a fertile field for the future development of alcohol-related cardiomyopathy.

Alcohol exerts its devastating effect in several ways: First, it acts as a poison, having a direct toxic effect on our heart muscle. Second, a rare contributing factor is the presence of other cardiotoxic substances, such as cobalt, in alcoholic beverages. In the past, cobalt was added to some beers as a foam stabilizer, resulting in cardiac dysfunction in some individuals. A third and interesting accomplice is the malnutrition that often occurs with alcohol abuse—with thiamin and other essential nutrients often depleted in patients consuming large quantities of alcohol. This nutrient depletion most definitely plays a part in the development of a cardiomyopathy.

The good news is that withdrawal of alcohol may, in fact, reverse heart muscle dysfunction. For this reason, I recommend that my heart failure patients avoid all alcoholic beverages.

Before moving on to the hypertrophic cardiomyopathies, I must make one further point about the psychological management of these patients.

Recently, I cared for a 60-year-old man diagnosed with dilated cardiomyopathy. The patient suffered from diabetes, but was otherwise in excellent health. His one symptom was extremely mild shortness of breath, which occurred only with very vigorous exercise. Otherwise, he was active, vibrant, and quite content. The patient was referred to me for an angiogram to eliminate a possible diagnosis of severe underlying coronary disease. His catheterization revealed the presence of only mild coronary disease but severely diminished heart muscle function. After his angiogram, I spoke with the patient, his wife, and his son, discussing future plans and expectations. When asked about the possibility of dying, I had to inform him that his disease did, in fact, have certain clear risks. Because we do not know for certain what may befall an *individual* patient with this disorder, I also felt it infinitely more beneficial to stress the positive. Thus, I spent a good deal of time reinforcing the fact that none of us knows how long he or she will live. This patient may very well live a full and complete life. I have numerous other DCM patients who have done so. My belief is that it is imperative to try to foster a positive mental outlook in all ailments but perhaps mostly in those with variable outcomes such as dilated cardiomyopathies.

In addition to the standard medication for DCM, I advised a natural regimen including essential fatty acids, antioxidants, coenzyme Q-10, and L-carnitine. I do not have a long-term follow-up on this patient to share with you, but I do have many other patients with similar forms of heart disease who continue to live long and productive lives.

Hypertrophic Cardiomyopathy

We've only recently begun to understand hypertrophic cardiomyopathy (HCM), a disease in which the heart muscle inappropriately thickens. Nonetheless we have learned that several forms of hypertrophic cardiomyopathies exist, involving various segments of the heart muscle. In Japan, there is a form which afflicts the tip of the heart—called "apical hypertrophic cardiomyopathy"—affecting one-quarter of all Japanese HCM patients. Fortunately, this disorder usually has a benign outcome; patients commonly have limited symptoms and nearly normal life expectancies.

Most patients with HCM have no symptoms. When symptoms appear, however, the most common is shortness of breath, affecting 90 percent of symptomatic patients. Chest pain occurs in three-quarters of symptomatic patients, while fatigue and lightheadedness are less common. Typically, those with symptoms will feel them intensify when exerting themselves. One of the most ominous signs in hypertrophic cardiomyopathy exists in children who faint. Fainting ("syncope") in a child with hypertrophic cardiomyopathy augurs a possible, future, sudden cardiac death.

This terrifying possibility must be taken very seriously, with beta blockers as the first line of therapy. When beta blockers don't work, implantable cardioverter defibrillators (ICDs) are often implanted under the skin. Like pacemakers, ICDs constantly survey the heart's rhythm. Additionally, they deliver shocks when required for rhythm realignment.

In adult patients whose heart muscles are so thickened that they develop obstruction to blood flow as it exits the left ventricle, implanting a permanent pacemaker may result in a significant reduction in symptoms. This group of patients, however, is limited, representing only 10 percent of hypertrophic cardiomyopathy patients.

TABLE 18
Causes of Heart Failure in Children

Along with HCM, there are other causes of heart failure in children. These conditions are very rare, particularly in the United States. A number of them are caused by organisms that don't live in North America. When they occur, however, they are extremely serious and need to be treated immediately.

Cause	Disease Produced
Viral myocarditis: coxsackie and rubella viruses	• Most common causes of myocarditis in newborns.
Trypanosomal myocarditis: *Trypanosoma cruzi*	• This myocarditis is rare in the United States, but endemic in South America. The infection can take 30 years to manifest as myocarditis. Also called "Chaga's disease."
Obstructive cardiomyopathy	• HOCM: very rare in the United States.
Glycogen storage deficiency	• This enzyme deficiency results in an increase of glycogen in the heart, which results in congestive heart failure.
Infantile beri-beri	• This form of heart failure resulting from vitamin B_1 deficiency occurs most commonly in Southeast Asia and Africa.
Kawasaki disease: (mucocutaneous lymph node syndrome)	• This syndrome, which can cause fever, rash, fissured lips, strawberry tongue, and a late coronary insufficiency, is thought to be caused by a virus. It is seen in the United States.

In patients who continue to suffer symptoms even with medications and electronic pacing of their heartbeats, surgery to relieve the obstruction to blood flow (by removing a portion of the heart muscle) can sometimes be performed. This form of surgery provides patients with excellent results by improving symptoms over many years of follow-up.

Now that you understand the various causes of heart muscle dysfunction that can lead to heart failure, let's discuss the treatment of patients with congestive heart failure.

Treating Congestive Heart Failure

When treating a patient with congestive heart failure, the physician has two goals: to decrease the patient's suffering and to prolong his or her life. Until the 1980s, treatment strategies were geared mainly toward reducing symptoms, as there were limited data demonstrating prolongation of life with the medical management of heart failure patients. Over the past twenty years or so, however, there have been numerous studies evaluating the life-expanding roles of various medicinal agents. We will now discuss the treatment of this disorder in terms of improving symptoms and extending life.

Using diuretics, those substances which enhance elimination of water and salt from the body (by more frequent urination), is an excellent way to reduce symptoms in chronic congestive heart failure patients. In fact, diuretics are the mainstay of therapy. Unfortunately, one of their side effects includes a pertubation in the body's electrolytes—the minerals sodium, potassium, magnesium, and chloride. Patients being treated with these drugs should pay careful attention to mineral intake and have frequent laboratory assessments of their magnesium and potassium levels.

Digitalis, a pharmaceutical derived from the foxglove plant, has other benefits for symptomatic heart failure patients. Although digitalis has been steeped in controversy for the past 100 years, recent studies show it to be effective for improving symptoms in patients with weakened heart muscle function who also suffer from symptoms of congestive heart failure. In fact, two clinical trials, PROVED and RADIANCE, demonstrated that withdrawal of Digoxin, a form of digitalis, from heart failure patients worsened their symptoms.

Table 19
Conventional Treatment of Congestive Heart Failure

Treatment	Action	Potential Side Effects
Diuretics: Lasix, Demadex	Help eliminate water and salt from the body.	• May precipitate gout. • May impair glucose control in diabetics. • May perturb the balance of minerals: potassium, magnesium, sodium, and chloride.

Table 19 (Continued)
Conventional Treatment of Congestive Heart Failure

Digitalis: Digoxin	This derivative of the fox-glove plant has been shown to help patients with heart failure over the last 100 years.	• Abrupt withdrawal can worsen symptoms. • Can accumulate in kidney failure, leading to heart rhythm disturbances.
Nitrovasodilators (Isordil)	These drugs dilate the veins.	• Headache. • Decreased blood pressure. • Lightheadedness.
ACE inhibitors (angiotensin converting enzyme inhibitors): Accupril, Monopril Vasotec, captopril	These drugs dilate the arteries, and are also beneficial to patients with leaky heart valves.	• A dry, hacking cough.
Beta blockers: especially Coreg	These drugs help congestive heart failure patients, but the mechanism by which they accomplish this is still being delineated.	• Can increase triglycerides. • Can decrease heart-protective HDL cholesterol. • Can cause difficulty breathing and precipitate asthma attacks. • Can cause leg pain or sensitivity to cold in patients whose arteries in the legs are blocked. • Hair loss. • Depression. • Fatigue. • Nightmares.
The "Batista operation"	This type of surgery was pioneered by the famous South American surgeon, Dr. Batista. It reconstructs the heart and, by cutting out a piece, makes it smaller and more geometrically sound.	• All heart surgery is associated with a certain level of risk, but this surgery generally achieves good results.

A third category of drugs beneficial in treating congestive heart failure patients includes the nitrovasodilators. These drugs (such as Isordil) dilate the venous system and are beneficial not only for reducing symptoms but also for prolonging life. The ACE (angiotensin converting enzyme) inhibitors—which dilate the arterial system—although extremely beneficial at prolonging life, have demonstrated only limited applicability in treating congestive heart failure symptoms. Nonetheless, there is a special, small group of patients with heart failure—those with leaky aortic and mitral valves—who benefit symptomatically from ACE inhibitors. These patients have been shown to experience not only an improvement in their symptoms, but also a less frequent progression of symptoms when taking ACE inhibitors.

Several studies have found that drug treatment of heart failure patients results in reduced mortality. The VHeFT Trial, one of the first to prove the point, utilized both hydralazine (an arterial dilator) and Isordil (a venous dilator). In this study, researchers documented a clear reduction in mortality with the combined use of these agents. The CONSENSUS trial also exhibited a 40 percent improvement in mortality in patients with severe congestive heart failure when taking enalapril (Vasotec).

The SAVE trial, which focused on asymptomatic patients with previous heart attacks, demonstrated a decrease both in mortality and disease progression. Patients in the SAVE study were treated with captopril, an ACE inhibitor. Its importance in treating this group of patients, even in the absence of any symptoms, was clearly demonstrated. Thus, if you are a patient with evident heart failure or a weakened heart muscle and can tolerate an ACE inhibitor, you should be on it. If you are not taking this medicine, please discuss this with your doctor.

A dry, hacking cough is a common and troublesome side effect of the ACE inhibitors. This symptom appears in 5 percent of patients treated with these drugs, and when it develops, it is often necessary to stop the ACE inhibitors. Fortunately, a new category of agents, very similar to the angiotensin converting enzyme inhibitors, has been developed. This drug class includes medications such as Cozaar and Diovan. It is believed that they, too, will provide mortality benefits in patients suffering from cardiomyopathies and congestive heart failure.

Although a "best" dose has not been established for many medications, the studies that showed mortality benefits from the following agents utilized these regimens: (1) 50 mg of captopril were administered three times a day; (2) 10 mg of enalapril (Vasotec) were administered twice a day; and (3) 10 mg of lisinopril were given once a day. It is not clear, however, how administering higher or lower dosages may affect outcomes.

Beta blockers represent a category of drugs previously considered anathema in patients with cardiomyopathies or congestive heart failure. In fact, beta agonists—the opposite of beta blockers—are beneficial in treating patients with acute heart failure. In patients with chronic heart failure, however, beta blockers have recently been shown to be beneficial; they decrease mortality and diminish symptom development. Although numerous theories attempt to explain the benefits of beta blockers, how they exert their beneficial effects remains a mystery.

Milrinone, a phosphodiesterase inhibitor, is another oral agent studied as a treatment for severe heart failure. Phosphodiesterase inhibitors are drugs which increase the heart muscle's ability to contract. In the PROMISE Trial, a 53 percent *increase* in mortality was documented in patients treated with this drug. In effect, the PROMISE Trial destroyed the "promise" of the phosphodiesterase inhibitor's usefulness in chronic heart failure patients. This trial reinforced a valuable lession in medicine—just because something "makes sense" does not guarantee its utility. Although it appeared that milrinone would save the lives of CHF patients, the opposite actually results.

Acute congestive heart failure represents an entirely different story. In this setting, the patient appears with a dramatic exacerbation of symptoms, which frequently results from a change in therapy, such as a medication change or perhaps a dietary indiscretion (i.e., the patient suddenly starts eating potato chips and hot dogs). Rhythm disturbances such as atrial fibrillation and slow heart rhythms can also result in a dramatic deterioration and acute heart failure. Other disorders such as infections, and physical or emotional stress, can precipitate acute heart failure. When it occurs, this syndrome is, of course, treated initially by removing the underlying cause. If this intervention is insufficient in returning patients to their baselines, they often require hospitalization and treatment with more potent drugs. When patients are hospitalized for acute heart failure, physicians usually employ intravenous forms of diuretics, as they possess greater potency and effectiveness than the oral forms. The phosphodiesterase inhibitors can also be safely used in an intravenous form as a effective, short-term means of treating heart failure. Dobutamine, another intravenous agent that acts by stimulating the beta receptors, promotes dilatation of blood vessels and increased inotropy (squeeze of the heart). This drug is often used for three to five days in order to bring the patient back to baseline—to get him "back on his feet."

When drugs fail in the treatment of congestive heart failure, more aggressive approaches come to the fore, including cardiac transplantation itself. Through better immunosuppressive drugs, transplantation has achieved vastly improved success. Presently, there is over a 60 percent survival rate six years out from heart transplantation. Unfortunately, because of a limited supply of heart donors, the average waiting time for a heart is eighteen months. As a result of the delay in treatment, 10 to 20 percent of patients waiting for a heart die suddenly, usually from a heart rhythm disturbance. It is a pity that the source of hearts is so limited; that more people do not agree to become organ donors. Nevertheless, the number of transplants being performed annually is increasing steadily, and in 1994 over 30,000 transplants had been performed in 257 centers.

As an alternative to heart transplantation, the famous South American surgeon Dr. Batista developed a procedure in which a portion of the heart muscle is actually removed, resulting in an improvement in the heart muscle's ability to function. This procedure is currently in its infancy, so we do not have long-term results or good follow-up of large numbers of patients, but I feel that it will become more commonly utilized in the twenty-first century.

I also hope that integrative medicine will become one of the standards of care as we enter the new millennium. In this regard, let me share with you the story of Rabbi Rosenthal, a gentleman with heart failure, who required the integration of natural modalities into a standard treatment regimen in order to improve his life.

Rabbi Rosenthal was a 60-year-old gentleman who came to me several years ago after having a bypass operation at the Massachusetts General Hospital in Boston. This is an excellent institution evincing wonderful outcomes in the surgical treatment of heart disease. Rabbi Rosenthal, however, developed complications. His operation had used both of his mammary arteries, and as a result he developed a sternal wound infection postoperatively—in other words, his chest became infected and the breast bone died. The rabbi required extensive reconstructive plastic surgery to re-create an adequate chest wall out of muscles and skin. After spending months in the hospital, he was discharged and ultimately returned to work as a temple rabbi.

Shortly after moving to Florida, the rabbi developed recurrent angina. I performed an angiogram and an angioplasty, and inserted a stent to his right coronary artery, relieving many of his symptoms. Unfortunately, he developed congestive heart failure as a result of a weakened heart muscle and a leaky mitral valve. The rabbi was treated with all the standard drugs that we have just discussed: Digoxin, diuretics, and ACE inhibitors. His symptoms persisted, however, necessitating multiple hospital admissions for acute heart failure.

The rabbi was becoming increasingly frustrated and angry. The vital life he had lived was slipping through his fingers. In Oriental terms, his *chi* was dissipating.

I suggested to the rabbi that we attempt to incorporate some more natural elements into his drug regimen. With a blend of stifled skepticism and cautious optimism, he agreed. I added the following items to the rabbi's regimen: coenzyme Q-10 to improve energy formation by the mitochondria; L-carnitine to increase fatty acid entry into the mitochondria, where it would be used for energy production; essential fatty acids for their possible reduction of rhythm disturbances; thiamin for its benefit in heart failure patients; magnesium for its vasodilating capabilities; L-arginine for its vasodilating capabilities and documented improvement in heart failure patients and a potent multimineral, multivitamin supplement as well.

The rabbi rebounded and made a complete recovery. He is now back to his vital self, lecturing, teaching, helping, and most impressively, smiling. The rabbi was reborn, and it was nature that led to his rebirth.

CHAPTER 8

Valvular Heart Disease: Disorders of "Too Much" and "Too Little"

Valvular heart disease prompts some of the most dramatic interventions in medicine, such as valve replacement with metal devices or pieces of pig hearts. Symptoms can develop suddenly, and can be life-threatening. Although supplements can help thin the blood and energize the heart muscle in patients with valvular diseases, let's remember that these conditions can be killers, and generally require aggressive medical intervention with strong drugs or surgery, once symptoms appear.

Four valves separate the four chambers of our hearts. In discussing valvular heart disease, however, only the valves of the left side—the mitral and aortic valves—commonly present problems.

As a result of disease, each of the four valves can leak or narrow. A leaky valve is referred to as being "regurgitant" (or "insufficient"), while a narrowed valve is dubbed "stenotic."

Mitral Stenosis

In mitral stenosis, the mitral valve (which separates the left atrium from the left ventricle) narrows. With its smaller than normal opening, the valve impedes blood flow from the left atrium to the left ventricle. When significantly narrowed (stenosed), a series of symptoms often develop, including shortness of breath—caused by the backup of blood into the lungs. If this sounds familiar to you, it should, since patients with congestive heart failure also suffer from the same underlying problem.

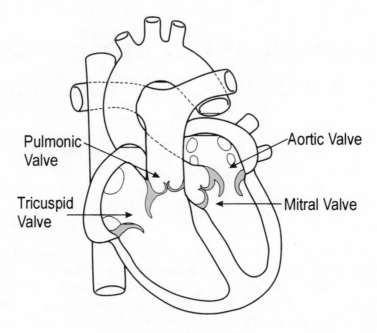

Pulmonic Valve

Aortic Valve

Tricuspid Valve

Mitral Valve

Heart Valves

A persistent cough can also be a troubling symptom of mitral stenosis. Other patients cough up blood (hemoptysis). The blood can be either excessive or slight, as with patients who produce a pink, frothy sputum. Chest pain, similar to that of angina, can also occur when the mitral valve narrows, even in the absence of other heart disease.

In general, these symptoms do not appear until a patient's valve area has substantially narrowed. A normal mitral valve orifice (opening) is between 4 and 6 cm^2, approximately the size of a walnut (5 centimeters is about 2 inches). When the area narrows to less than 2 cm^2, the diagnosis is clear: mild mitral stenosis (narrowing).

Initially, a very slight blood pressure gradient develops across the mitral valve. As the valve area diminishes, a large gradient becomes necessary to maintain adequate blood flow from the left atrium to the left ventricle. Like a garden hose with a kink in it, pressure builds up behind the damaged valve—the kink in the hose—so it is higher behind the kink (or the malfunctioning valve) than it is in front of it. In its worst form "severe" mitral stenosis results, and these patients can develop serious symptoms. Conditions that cause increased heart rates and cardiac output generally worsen symptoms. Because the body can no longer compensate for the valve's dysfunction, a fever, overactive thyroid, and any exercise (conditions which increase the heart rate) can lead to a downward spiral.

Rheumatic heart disease is the commonest cause of mitral stenosis. (Other, very rare causes include congenital heart disease, carcinoid, lupus, and rheumatoid arthritis.) When rheumatic fever strikes, it can affect all components of a mitral valve. Indeed, it may result in a gradual narrowing of the valve, with symptoms taking ten or more years to develop.

A fascinating but poorly understood fact is that mitral stenosis develops much more rapidly in tropical climates than it does in temperate zones. Because of this, the age at which mitral valve stenosis develops is significantly younger in the tropics than it is in temperate regions.

When patients develop *symptomatic* mitral stenosis, they initially receive medical therapy. Antibiotics are given to prevent future bouts of rheumatic fever, and they are provided prophylactically to prevent bacteria from devouring a deformed heart valve. When shortness of breath is an issue, diuretics can eliminate excess fluid from the lungs.

Those patients with mitral valve stenosis who develop an abnormal heart rhythm, or "atrial fibrillation," require Digoxin and occasionally beta blockers to minimize their symptoms. (It has also been found that beta-blocker therapy can significantly improve exercise capacity in such patients.) When atrial fibrillation occurs, patients must take the blood thinner Coumadin—since mitral stenosis patients experiencing atrial fibrillation represent one of the highest risk groups for future strokes.

Surgery with either valve repair or replacement becomes necessary when patients develop symptoms and their mitral valve areas have narrowed to less than 1 to 1.5 cm^2. Additionally, those patients who suffer from emboli—blood clots which have traveled to various parts of the body—should be operated on to decrease their risk of future emboli. With valve repair, the current mortality risk stands at 1–3 percent, with an excellent five-year survival rate—greater than 90 percent. We must remember, however, that this form of surgery is palliative; it is not curative. The valve remains abnormal and it can narrow again (a process called "restenosis").

Mitral valve replacement—a riskier surgery—carries a higher mortality hazard of 3–8 percent. As a result, patients should opt for this procedure only when valve repair is not appropriate.

The least invasive approach to correct mitral stenosis physically involves "balloon mitral valvuloplasty," a procedure performed through the groin, like coronary angioplasty. A single or double balloon is passed through the mitral valve and then expanded, cracking the valve open and widening the size of the mitral valve orifice. The risk here is much lower than that of surgical interventions, with a mortality estimated at less than 1 percent. To undergo this procedure, however, patients must meet very strict echocardiographic criteria. When they do, success is common and surgery can be avoided.

Mitral Regurgitation

To understand mitral regurgitation (a leaky valve), we must examine the mitral valve apparatus. It is not a simple structure. The mitral valve contains four major components: the two leaflets that actually come together when the heart muscle contracts (in systole) and separate as the heart muscle relaxes (in diastole). The second component is the chordae tendineae, which attach the leaflets to the papillary muscles (the third component) that help to control the movement of the mitral valve leaflets themselves. The annulus, the fourth structure, is a ring to which the leaflets attach.

A defect in any one of these four components can result in significant mitral regurgitation. When an abnormality of the valve leaflets is the underlying cause, rheumatic heart disease is usually the culprit. It is interesting to note that this condition is more common in men than women, whereas mitral stenosis (narrowing) from rheumatic heart disease is more common in women than in men. We don't know why this is. Infections of and trauma to the leaflets are other, more unusual causes of mitral regurgitation.

An abnormality in the mitral valve annulus (the ring) is a fairly common cause of mitral regurgitation. The annulus is normally a soft, pliable structure that constricts as the heart muscle squeezes.

When it becomes calcified with age, a condition called MAC ("mitral annular calcification") results. This is extremely common and usually benign. There are some unusual cases, however, in which significant calcification can result in mitral regurgitation when the stiffened annulus fails to constrict properly as the rest of the heart squeezes. Patients with high blood pressure, diabetes, and kidney failure are particularly prone to developing this problem. Other patients, like those with heart failure, can develop mitral regurgitation as their heart muscles dilate, expanding the mitral annulus and thus not allowing the leaflets to come together (coapt) properly.

An abnormality in the chordae tendineae can also occasionally cause mitral regurgitation. The chordae, fine string-like structures, can spontaneously break in a patient with mitral valve prolapse or rheumatic heart disease. I recently saw a patient who was completely asymptomatic and yet suffered from moderate to severe mitral regurgitation because of a spontaneously ruptured chordae tendineae. He is a fully active man and since he is asymptomatic, we are treating him conservatively, using ACE inhibitors and calcium channel blockers to ease the burden on his heart, and careful observation. This patient continues to exercise, and as long as he remains asymptomatic, he will be able to avoid the trauma of surgery. If, however, a future echocardiogram demonstrates a worsening of his heart muscle's function, or if he develops significant symptoms, he will have to undergo valve repair to prevent heart muscle failure.

The fourth component of the mitral valve which, when diseased, can lead to mitral regurgitation is its papillary muscles. Two papillary muscles connect the chordae tendineae to the mitral valve leaflets. These muscles are extremely vulnerable to conditions in which their blood supply is jeopardized. Therefore, in patients suffering from coronary disease, papillary muscles can become dysfunctional and even rupture in rare—but devastating—circumstances.

If you are a patient suffering from mitral regurgitation or from any of the other ailments discussed here, you must keep in mind the fact that each of these disorders possesses a spectrum of illness ranging from very mild to very severe. With mitral regurgitation, for example, patients with mild leaks can remain asymptomatic for their entire lives. These patients rarely develop severe mitral regurgitation. Once symptoms develop, however, it can be too late to perform corrective surgery. If you have such a condition, be sure to visit your doctor frequently and to have yearly echocardiograms.

When treating mitral regurgitation with medicine, drugs called "afterload reducing agents" are our most important tools. They dilate the arterial bed, making it easier for the left ventricle to pump blood forward, which decreases the amount of blood that "regurgitates," streaming backward into the left atrium.

ACE inhibitors—such agents—are extremely effective at decreasing the symptoms of mitral regurgitation and have been shown to prolong survival in these patients. Although Digoxin and diuretics are also beneficial, they have not been shown to prolong life in these patients.

Also helpful are the herbs hawthorn, a "natural" ACE inhibitor, and khella, a "natural" calcium channel blocker. In regard to hawthorn, I generally prescribe 100–900 mg hawthorn leaf/flower extract daily, taken in two or three divided doses. As for khella, 100 mg of 12 percent Khellin can be taken three times daily.

When medicine is inadequate and surgery becomes necessary, valves can be either reconstructed or replaced. In young patients with pliable valves, reconstruction is often the treatment of choice. Older or sicker patients usually require mitral valve replacements. One problem with mitral valve replacements is that heart muscles can actually deteriorate after natural mitral valves are removed from the heart. Nonetheless, preservation of the annular-chordal and papillary muscle connection can actually maintain heart muscle function, even after removal of the natural mitral valve. Therefore, it is current practice for surgeons to try to preserve this apparatus, even when replacing mitral valves, to ensure excellent heart muscle function.

In determining who should undergo mitral valve surgery for mitral regurgitation, two assessments are primary: symptoms and heart size. First, patients who have significant symptoms and severe mitral regurgitation should undergo surgery. Second, even those patients who are asymptomatic should undergo surgery when they show deterioration of their left ventricular function, which can be seen on routine echocardiography. Over the last several years, we have been performing surgery on these patients more aggressively, as we have found that waiting too long can result in irreparable damage to the left heart.

Mitral valve prolapse (MVP, also known as Barlow syndrome), a disorder that can involve any of the components of the mitral valve, deserves special attention. As its name implies, mitral valve prolapse occurs when the valve leaflets bow back (i.e., prolapse) into the left atrium during ventricular systole. Happily, the most common outcome here is *nothing*. As it is such a prevalent condition, however, affecting 3 to 5 percent of the general population, and 5 to 10 percent of all women, and because of the fact that a small segment of mitral valve prolapse patients does develop troubling symptoms, the disorder has taken on ominous, even mysterious characteristics. Additionally, prior to the development of Perloff's criteria for diagnosing mitral valve prolapse—using echocardiography and physical examination—the disorder was grossly over-diagnosed.

Although most patients never experience any symptoms from this condition, and it exists in isolation in the vast majority of patients, there really are some extremely fascinating findings which can be associated with it. For instance, there is a higher incidence of bony abnormalities like a misshapen chest wall (pectus excavatum) or an abnormal twisting of the spine (scoliosis) in patients with mitral valve prolapse. The autonomic nervous system can occasionally be out of synch in MVP patients, resulting in low blood pressure upon standing up (postural hypotension), easy fatigability, and palpitations. Ministrokes, or TIAs (transient ischemic attacks), are also slightly more common in mitral valve prolapse patients. Why? Perhaps it's due to tiny little emboli (blood clots) that float off the abnormal valve and travel to the brain. Aspirin is probably the best drug to treat TIAs with, but occasionally even Coumadin is needed.

Some MVP patients suffer from chest discomfort that can resemble angina. This pain is often associated with palpitations. When patients are troubled by these symptoms, beta blockers become the mainstay of pharmaceutical drug therapy. Those rare patients who experience fainting or near-fainting spells should undergo Holter monitoring or stress test evaluation to determine whether they are susceptible to significant rhythm disturbances. When a dangerous disturbance is uncovered, electrophysiological studies are indicated, as there is an extremely low, but real, increased risk of sudden cardiac death in a *small* subset of these patients.

Patients with mitral regurgitation associated with this disorder must be followed closely to ensure that they do not develop *signifi-*

cant mitral regurgitation. Currently, mitral valve prolapse is the leading cause of valve deformities in those patients undergoing mitral valve replacements to correct mitral regurgitation. In mitral valve prolapse, the general prognosis for regurgitation is actually excellent, as only 15 percent of patients have a meaningful progression over a fifteen-year follow-up period.

You can see that mitral valve prolapse is a very common but generally extremely benign condition. It is only the rare and unusual patient who suffers a serious outcome from this disorder. With regard to a natural approach to MVP, coenzyme Q-10 and magnesium are the best natural means to diminish its symptoms, and they are very safe to use in this setting.

Aortic Valve Disease

The aortic valve, as you now know, is an extremely important structure: It is the "good" blood's final barrier between the heart and the rest of the body. When this valve grows defective, therefore, each of our organs is jeopardized.

Aortic Stenosis

In the case of aortic stenosis, a narrowing of the valve limits the flow of blood from the left ventricle into the aorta. As the constriction progresses, the left ventricle must struggle with greater intensity to force blood through the shrinking orifice. This can result in pressures within the left ventricle exceeding 300 mm of mercury!

Although a congenitally abnormal aortic valve can cause this condition, a more common culprit is the wear and tear of aging, which is referred to as degenerative or senile calcific aortic stenosis. With age, a gradual deposition of calcium along the aortic valve results in a stiffening, thickening, and overall reduction in the flexibility and movement of this valve. Two coronary risk factors, diabetes mellitus and high cholesterol, are also known to predispose one to senile calcific aortic stenosis. The course of this disorder is usually insidious, with a gradually progressive narrowing occurring over many years. Patients are commonly free of any symptoms until severe aortic stenosis strikes. The presence of symptoms implies the need for surgery, since there are no medications which can effectively treat aortic stenosis. The instant an adult patient develops the symptoms of aortic stenosis, his or her prognosis becomes limited. There is no natural approach to treating this disorder—this patient absolutely needs surgery.

The three symptoms that augur doom in these patients are chest pain (angina), fainting (syncope), and congestive heart failure. Their 50 percent survival rates are five years, three years, and two years respectively (in the absence of surgical intervention). Angina, the least ominous of these three symptoms, occurs because of an increasing need for oxygen due to an overactive and thickening heart muscle. Fainting can result from several causes. Heart rhythm disturbances (such as atrioventricular block and transient ventricular fibrillation) can precipitate fainting here, as can exercise. As we exercise, the blood vessels supplying skeletal muscles tend to dilate, placing increasing demands on our hearts to pump more and more blood to the working muscles. In the setting of a severely narrowed aortic valve, blood pressure can drop precipitously during exercise, causing patients to faint.

Congestive heart failure, the most ominous of the three aortic stenosis symptoms, usually develops as the thickened heart muscle begins to fail—unable to continue its struggle against an immobile opponent, the narrowed and hardened aortic valve.

Echocardiography is the best noninvasive means of diagnosing significant aortic stenosis. Once symptoms have occurred in the patient with severe aortic stenosis, he or she should undergo a cardiac catheterization and an aortic valve replacement. Unfortunately, valve repair is ineffective. Mortality during aortic valve replacement surgery ranges between 1 and 8 percent, depending upon the relative illness of the patient.

Balloon valvuloplasty, as described in the mitral stenosis section, is not nearly so effective in patients with degenerative calcific aortic stenosis. In fact, it is currently almost never used. At times, however, children with congenital aortic stenosis can benefit from the procedure.

As with cases of mitral and aortic regurgitation, aortic stenosis is now being more aggressively treated with early surgical intervention. Years ago, we delayed surgery until the last possible moment. Although it is still considered useful to delay any surgery, we no longer wait quite so long, thus avoiding possible irreparable damage to our heart muscles, or even worse, death.

Aortic Regurgitation

When the aortic valve is leaky, blood courses backward from the aorta through the valve and back into the left ventricle during diastole, the time of ventricular relaxation. This "overload" results in a gradual enlarging of the left ventricle. In fact, the left ventricle can, at times, become so huge that it seems to resemble a cow's heart or *cor bovinum*. The object of therapy, of course, is to avoid the development of *cor bovinum*.

Aortic regurgitation is caused by either a widening (dilatation) of the aortic root—that part of the aorta in which the valve resides—or a disorder of the valve itself. As in the case of mitral regurgitation (in which the mitral valve leaflets fail to meet and form a good seal), when the aortic root dilates excessively, the aortic valve cannot close tightly enough to prevent blood from leaking back into the left ventricle. In patients with pure aortic regurgitation, over half also suffer from aortic root disease—the actual cause of their problem. High blood pressure is probably the most common cause of aortic root dilatation but other factors such as an age-related expansion of the aortic root, syphilitic involvement of the aortic root, and ulcerative colitis can also predispose to aortic root disease and subsequent aortic regurgitation.

When the valve itself is the primary culprit in aortic regurgitation, a variety of disorders can carry the blame, including lupus, Crohn's disease, rheumatic heart disease, and rheumatoid arthritis. Certainly, the symptom to fear most with aortic regurgitation is congestive heart failure. When a patient with severe aortic regurgitation develops heart failure, he or she has a 50 percent two-year survival rate in the absence of surgery. Contrast this with a 50 percent survival rate at ten years in the *asymptomatic* patient with severe aortic regurgitation!

These asymptomatic patients are usually treated with vasodilators, such as nifedipine, which can delay the need for surgery. Frequent echocardiograms and clinical assessments to safeguard their stability, however, are necessary as well.

Although studies have yet to be done on hawthorn, khella, magnesium, coenzyme Q-10, and L-carnitine I believe they are helpful to patients with aortic regurgitation. How do they work? By dilating blood vessels, hawthorn, khella, and magnesium can decrease the excess burden on the heart. Simultaneously, L-carnitine and coenzyme Q-10 may improve the heart's ability to contract (beat) against the blood volume overload that's inherent in aortic regurgitation.

Unfortunately, when patients with severe aortic regurgitation develop any symptoms of heart failure, or deterioration of their left ventricle, surgery is our only recourse. To avoid possible permanent weakening of the left heart valve, we also like to operate before dysfunction develops in the left ventricle.

Abnormalities of the Right Heart Valves

Replacing either of the right heart valves, the tricuspid and pulmonic valves, is now quite uncommon. Tricuspid stenosis (TS), resulting from rheumatic heart disease, can occasionally be severe enough, however, to require valve replacement. Patients with severe TS can suffer from the effects of a low cardiac output, with fatigue, lethargy, and decreased appetite. They can also develop signs of right heart valve failure, with swelling in their legs and belly. At times, these patients require surgery.

When a valve replacement is needed in the tricuspid position, it's not possible to replace it with a mechanical valve; only a tissue valve can be used. Mechanical valves tend to have a prohibitively high rate of thrombosis (clotting off) in this location.

Tricuspid regurgitation (TR) can occasionally become severe in patients with dilated right ventricles caused by coexisting mitral valve disease. Death of the right ventricle as a result of a substantial heart attack can also result in severe TR. Again in most cases, tricuspid regurgitation is very well tolerated, with surgery rarely called for. When surgery is a must, a ring as opposed to a valve replacement, is often the surgeon's first choice. I recall from my days at Bellevue an interesting group of patients with severe tricuspid regurgitation: drug addicts with tricuspid valve endocarditis. Occasionally, an intravenous drug abuser would present with such a grave infection involving the tricuspid valve that a significant valve leak would result. When the magnitude of the infection overwhelmed antibiotic therapy, surgeons would sometimes remove the valve without replacing it, leaving the patient without a tricuspid valve. Remarkably, these patients did very well, tolerating the absence for months on end. Only when the patient became healthier and free of infection would surgeons attempt to replace the valve.

Pulmonic Valve Disease

Pulmonic valve disorders are the rarest of valve problems, and usually represent congenital anomalies. When congenital pulmonic stenosis occurs, balloon valvuloplasty is often the treatment of choice.

Cardiac Valve Prostheses

Nearly forty years have passed since surgeons first successfully replaced a valve in a human being. Since then, the tremendous technological advances in valve prostheses have been complemented by the research evaluating them. Currently, there are two major categories of prosthetic valves: mechanical and bioprosthetic (tissue).

The first mechanical valves that were developed also have the greatest durability. The Starr-Edwards, or caged-ball, valve has lasted over twenty-five years in some patients without requiring reoperation. Nonetheless, this valve is extremely bulky and carries with it a higher risk of embolic events than do the more modern varieties—the sleeker tilting disc mechanical valves. The St. Jude, the prototypical tilting disc valve, is the most widely used of all mechanical valves. Less bulky than the Starr-Edwards valve, it is thus more applicable in the treatment of childhood valve disorders. This valve (as seen on page 133) incorporates two half-moon discs which open and close as the heart beats.

The need for long-term anticoagulation with Coumadin is the major drawback of all mechanical valves. When patients with mechanical valves are not anticoagulated, they have a three- to sixfold increase in the risk of embolic events. A particularly dramatic and devastating consequence of *not* anticoagulating patients with these valves can be the abrupt clotting off of the entire valve, most often leading to death.

I am often asked whether "natural" blood thinners—like ginkgo, vitamin E, garlic, or the Omega-3 oils—can be used instead of Coumadin. The answer is *no*. To date, there have been no studies documenting the efficacy of these substances. If patients wish to add these substances to their Coumadin, I feel they can, but only under the watchful eye of a physician.

This clotting problem, which led to exploring alternative valve prostheses that would not require potent blood thinners, has prompted the development of a new class of tisssue valves. Tissue taken from pig heart valves, the porcine heterografts, for example, have been used since 1965 for treating mitral and aortic valve disorders. Although it's recommended that some patients (especially those receiving porcine mitral valves) be anticoagulated for the first three months following surgery, long-term anticoagulation is not necessary. There is a small group of patients who have had prior emboli (blood clots), a history of atrial fibrillation, or a clot noted in their left atrium, for whom, even with porcine mitral valve replacements, long-term anticoagulation remains necessary.

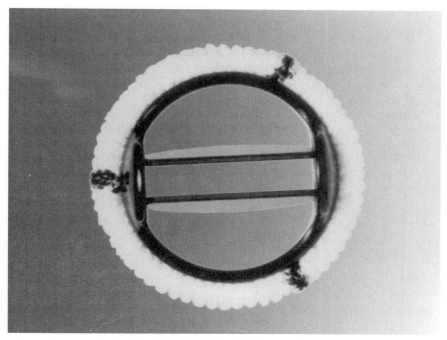

St. Jude Mechanical Heart Valve

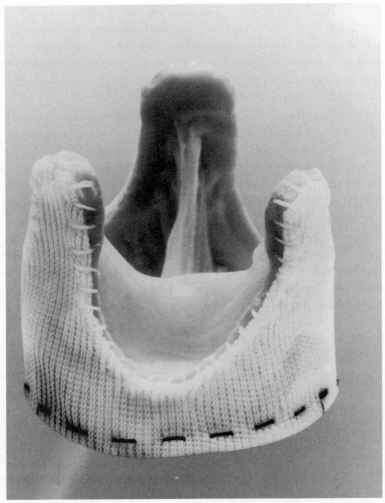

St. Jude Bioprosthetic Valve

On the downside, porcine valve replacements do not last all that long, requiring replacement within ten years of surgery in over one-third of cases. Because young patients are particularly prone to a rapid deterioration of their tissue valves, they generally require mechanical valve replacements.

Another kind of tissue valve, the homograft valve, is removed from cadavers. Homograft valves, used predominantly in the aortic position, also allow for improved blood flow beyond their mechanical and even porcine forms. With modern techniques of preservation, these valves have become extremely effective. Their major disadvantage is their limited availability.

The final and most captivating of the tissue valve replacements is the "pulmonary autograft." In this operation, highly skilled surgeons delicately remove the patient's own pulmonary valve and place it in the aortic position. They then use a tissue valve as a pulmonary valve replacement. This surgery is extremely complicated and only the most highly trained surgeons are capable of doing it. Because of this, it is generally performed at only very specialized centers and reserved for valve replacements in young adults.

General guidelines for choosing between mechanical and prosthetic valves in valve replacement surgery include the following:

- As mechanical valves have been shown to have better long-term results and even better survival rates in some trials, they are the valves of choice in patients who can tolerate anticoagulation.
- When patients are poor candidates for long-term blood thinners—for instance, when they are noncompliant with their medications, have a tendency to bleed, or are over the age of 70 and thus prone to developing future bleeding tendencies—they should receive bioprosthetic valve replacements.
- Patients under the age of 40 requiring aortic valve replacements should give serious consideration to the use of pulmonary autografts. Once again, there are only a few surgeons who are expert in performing this particular operation and thus patients should research the center and the surgeon who will perform this delicate procedure.

Natural Regimens for Valvular Heart Disease

Although supplements are generally of less value in valvular heart disease than with other heart disorders, particular patients can use the following to help with their conditions:

- Hawthorn extract for aortic and mitral regurgitation
- Coenzyme Q-10 for aortic and mitral regurgitation and aortic stenosis to improve heart muscle function

- Magnesium for mitral stenosis to help limit atrial fibrillation
- Omega-3 fatty acids to prevent rhythm disturbances in all disorders
- L-carnitine to improve heart muscle function in all valve disorders
- L-arginine to vasodilate and possibly improve heart function in mitral and aortic insufficiency

Patients with these conditions, however, should consult a physician who practices integrative medicine to determine the quantities and types of supplements they should add to their treatment regimen. Mr. William Murray, a feeble 86-year-old was being treated with powerful traditional medications for a multitude of cardiac ailments—valve disease, heart failure, coronary artery disease, and arrythmia.

Over six months, Mr. Murray became wheelchair-bound, experiencing neurological problems, most likely as a result of one of the powerful medicines being used to treat his heart rhythm disturbance. As doctors say, the patient was failing to thrive.

His wife called me in on consultation, hoping that I might be able to alter his medications and bring him back to a level of functioning that would make his remaining months or, hopefully, years more livable. Unfortunately, his traditional doctor had refused to eliminate any of his pharmaceutical agents, stating that they were necessary to sustain his life.

After evaluating Mr. Murray, I discussed a variety of options with him and his wife. One method of restoring quality of life involved discontinuing one of his anti-arrhythmic medications. This could be viewed by some as being tantamount to opening the windows of an armored vehicle while passing through a potentially hazardous territory. Although risky, it was not at all clear that stopping his medicine would definitely cause a life-threatening heart rhythm disturbance.

Mr. and Mrs. Murray both accepted the potential hazard of freedom from this medication. They also wished to try any natural approach possible. I prescribed a variety of supplements and herbs which would likely help his heart. As a baseline for him (as with all my patients), I recommended a powerful multivitamin, multimineral supplement with high-dose antioxidants. Additionally, I advised hawthorn extract for both his heart muscle function and potential improvement in his heart's electrical system. High-dose coenzyme Q-10 was used for his heart failure, and magnesium was added for his rhythm disturbance.

It has been nearly two years since I initiated this protocol, and Mr. Murray not only lives on, but functions on a much higher level than he would have had he continued his pharmaceutical drugs. I certainly do not know how long Mr. Murray will live, but I know that he and his wife have assumed responsibility for their lives and their health. They, not the medical profession, have determined the course they will take, and it has served them well.

A final concern for patients with abnormal heart valves is a potentially serious infection called subacute bacterial endocarditis (SBE). When your doctor informs you that you require antibiotics prior to undergoing dental procedures or other invasive and "unclean" procedures, it is because he or she is attempting to prevent an abnormal heart valve from becoming infected by bacteria invading the blood. During deep dental cleaning, for instance, you surely have noted the excessive bleeding that can occur as the dental hygienist strips away deep layers of plaque. Since the mouth is filled with bacteria, this poking and prodding can introduce numerous bugs into the bloodstream. An abnormal valve represents a cozy resting place for these bacteria. When too many bacteria settle on an abnormal heart valve, our bodies can no longer fight them off, and a valve infection may ensue. The antibiotics are prescribed to help prevent it.

Antibiotics are recommended before invasive procedures for patients with mitral valve prolapse who have audible murmurs or clear regurgitation (demonstrated on echocardiography). If, as your doctor examines you, he or she hears just a "click," then you probably have such a low chance of experiencing endocarditis that antibiotic prophylaxis is not advised. Other cardiac disorder (outlined in Table 20) also require antibiotic prophylaxis.

There have not yet been any good studies evaluating the use of antibiotic prophylaxis. However, since the antibiotics used for endocarditis prevention are generally harmless, their use is standard medical practice in various circumstances.

At the same time, it's certainly reasonable to use natural means of boosting the immune system to prevent bacterial infections from taking hold. Vitamin C, garlic, and the herb echinacea can all be used in conjunction with antibiotics to prevent bacterial endocarditis. They are by no means considered replacements for antibiotics.

TABLE 20
Cardiac Conditions for Which Endocarditis Prophylaxis May or May Not be Indicated

PROPHYLAXIS RECOMMENDED	PROPHYLAXIS NOT RECOMMENDED
• Prostetic cardiac valves, including bioprosthetic and homograph valves • Previous bacterial endocarditis, even in absence of heart disease • Surgically constructed systemic-pulmonary shunts • Most congenital cardiac malformations • Rheumatic acquired valvular dysfunction • Hypertropic cardiomyopathy • Mitral valve prolapse with valvular regurgitation	• Isolated secundum atrial septal defect • Surgical repair without residua beyond 6 monthos of: >secundum atrial septal defect >ventricular septal defect >patent ductus arteriosus • Previous coronary artery bypass surgery • Mitral valve prolapse without valvular regurgitation • Physiological, functional, or innocent heart murmurs • Previous Kawasaki disease or rheumatic fever without valvular dysfunction • Cardiac pacemakers and implanted defibrillators

Source: Dajani, A.S. et al. JAMA 264:2929–2922, 1990

Electrophysiology:
The Shocking Truth

More than a few physicians consider electrophysiology, itself a sub-specialty of cardiology, the most esoteric field in medicine. In fact, cardiology fellows across the country have been found hiding in remote parts of hospitals to avoid participating in electrophysiologic studies (EPS). Why, you might wonder? Well, there are many tedious stretches in EPSs—hours in the lab staring at minute, squiggly lines marching interminably across a TV screen. Subtle differences in the timing and shapes of the lines determine when the operator will make a dramatic decision, such as burning an area of the heart. Because of the nature of the field, computer nerds are often drawn to it. Somehow I, a computer illiterate, became interested in electrophysiology, completed extra training, and became board certified in the field. My mentor, Dr. David Rubin, was certainly a stimulating force, but there are other elements of this endeavor that are exciting, energetic, and, yes, electric. It is these fascinating parts of electrophysiology that I will explore with you to help you understand the electrical mishaps of the heart.

In the Appendix, I have provided a fairly comprehensive description of various electrical aberrations of the heart. You can either read the Appendix or simply use it as a reference should you or someone you care about develop a heart rhythm disorder. But for now, sit back and relax as we travel through the electrical circuitry of the heart.

The Basic Electrophysiology Study

The Florida sun beat brutally on Ramon Rodriguez as he bent down to set another tile on the roof. It was hot, but no hotter than any other July day in the sunshine state. At 20, he was one of the youngest and strongest of the migrant roofers. Like many of his co-workers, he had traveled from Guatemala to search for solid work. Roofing was good work. At each week's end, he was able to send money home to help his parents and younger siblings, who remained in Guatemala. In fact, on this particular July day, Ramon was feeling quite optimistic—until, without warning, out of nowhere, a train began charging from his chest into his neck. The pounding persisted. His head spun; he broke into a sweat, and sank limply to the roof. Fortunately, his friends were able to carry him safely to the ground, but he was unable to stand without assistance. The train incessantly roared through his body.

When the ambulance arrived at the emergency room, his heart was beating over 250 times a minute—about three times the rate of a normal heart. His blood pressure was a dangerously low 80/50; and although conscious, he was certainly not feeling himself. The emergency room physician did a thorough and extremely rapid evaluation of Ramon, and then appropriately sedated him in preparation for an electrical cardioversion. This is a procedure during which two paddles, or pads, are placed on the chest and back, and an electric current is sent through the body to restore the heart's normal rhythm. As Mr. Rodriguez fell asleep, the doctor gave the order. The nurse pushed the button and Mr. Rodriguez's back and chest lifted high off the stretcher. As he landed, the monitor clearly showed that the procedure had been successful. He was back in a normal rhythm—his heart beating peacefully at 60 beats per minute. Mr. Rodriguez awoke and, instantly aware of his restored rhythm, breathed a great sigh of relief.

As the only electrophysiologist on staff at our hospital, I was immediately called to evaluate Mr. Rodriguez. I spoke with the treating physician and evaluated the patient (and his EKG). It was clear that our patient had a condition called Wolff-Parkinson-White (WPW) syndrome. This is a congenital abnormality in which an extra circuit connects the upper and lower chambers of the heart. In a select group of patients whose circuits are able to conduct electrical impulses at an alarmingly dangerous rate, WPW can be a devastating problem. If atrial fibrillation were to occur (as it did with our young patient), the patient's life could be in jeopardy. Atrial fibrillation is a rapid, chaotic rhythm, emanating from the upper chambers of the heart (the atria). The atria quiver at nearly 500 times a minute during this rhythm. When "normal" hearts experience atrial fibrillation, the A-V node (the heart's natural filter) is able to protect the ventricles from experiencing such rapid rates. Because of this filter, the heart will usually beat at 100–150 beats per minute. In Mr. Rodriguez's case, the extra circuit in his heart bypassed the A-V node and allowed the ventricles to beat more than 250 times per minute. The result was low blood pressure, lightheadedness, and a close brush with death. Left unchecked, this condition would compromise Mr. Rodriguez's entire life. Soccer, his favorite pastime, would turn dangerous; roofing would be absolutely out of the question.

For Ramon Rodriguez to live a normal, carefree life, I advised him to undergo one of the few truly curative cardiac procedures—radio frequency (RF) ablation (or destruction) of his extra circuit (bypass tract). The procedure restores Mr. Rodriguez's electrical system to normal by using high-frequency radio waves to destroy the extra circuit that allowed his heart to beat so wildly.

Prior to this curative procedure, however, he would first undergo a diagnostic electrophysiologic study.

The electrophysiologic study (EPS), like a cardiac catheterization, requires the insertion of catheters into the heart. Thus, it is an invasive procedure and carries with it rare but present dangers. But let's return to Mr. Rodriquez.

Mr. Rodriguez is about to undergo an EPS. He is anxious. To make matters worse, he is ignorant. Although ignorance may be bliss in some circumstances, it is not when undergoing this or any other medical procedure. Ignorance allows Mr. Rodriguez to imagine only the most horrific possibilities. An uninformed patient is usually terrified. An informed patient is justifiably and realistically frightened. Thus, as I tell Mr. Rodriguez about an EPS, I also make him aware of any possible risks.

In terms of EPS, the catheters represent the greatest danger. In fewer than 1 out of 1,000 patients, the catheters can pierce the heart wall. This usually does not result in serious consequences. Occasionally, the sac around the heart (the pericardium) can be so engorged with blood that it requires drainage, using a needle and syringe. Rarely, the patient will require surgery. Even more rarely, the patient can die.

Other risks of the EPS include infections and bleeding problems, but they are also extremely rare. All in all, the EPS is an extraordinarily safe procedure; in fact, it is generally safer than a cardiac catheterization.

Now that Mr. Rodriguez understands the risks of the procedure, he should also know exactly what it entails.

Our patient will be slightly sedated with a small amount of Valium taken a half-hour before being wheeled into the EP lab. He'll be placed on his back on a narrow, hard table with a thin pad beneath him. The nurses will shave his groin area and wash it clean with Betadine (a cleansing solution). Then they'll drape a large cloth of paper over him from his chin down beyond his toes. As the room is kept cold because of the equipment, the nurses may also shroud him in blankets and towels beneath the sterile drape. To aid in positioning the catheters, the nurses will move the mobile table frequently during the procedure. Although a large fluoroscopy camera is located above and below the table, it's not smothering, so even claustrophobic patients will have no trouble here.

The doctor will numb the groin area with a fine needle and Lidocaine, which can feel like a bee sting, and place small tubes called sheaths within the femoral vein through punctures in the skin. No sutures are required. For his part, Mr. Rodriguez will feel pressure but no pain. The procedure is actually quite painless. Guided by the fluoroscope, the doctor will maneuver the catheters through the sheaths, into the femoral vein, and then backward and ultimately into the heart. Only when the catheters are placed in specific locations within the heart (which I'll discuss shortly) can the test begin.

Not all EP studies are the same, as indications for this test will vary. But, by way of example, I will describe a typical study.

The catheters are gently and carefully manipulated through the veins back toward the heart. They enter the right atrium first. The doctor places one catheter against the side wall of the atrium in close proximity to the natural pacemaker of the heart, the sinus node. A second catheter is placed across the tricuspid valve, its tip left lying between the right atrium and the right ventricle. The doctor then passes the third and final catheter across the tricuspid valve (at least in most studies), all the way into the right ventricle, at the tip of the heart called the apex.

In Mr. Rodriguez's case, things were different because he required an additional two catheters: an ablation catheter used to deliver radio-frequency energy to burn the extra pathway, and a monitoring catheter positioned in the coronary sinus (the vein that drains the heart).

The catheters have a dual function—they record energy emanating from the heart, and they deliver energy to the heart (i.e., they act as pacemakers). The first order of business is to evaluate the integrity of the heart's basic electrical circuitry. Are there any dramatic problems with the heart's electrical system? To begin our assessment, we make several simple measurements.

1. We measure how often the sinus node fires. This is the A-A interval, or the time between two beats of the heart. It gives us a sense of the health of the heart's natural pacemaker. Under normal circumstances, hearts beat between 60 and 100 times a

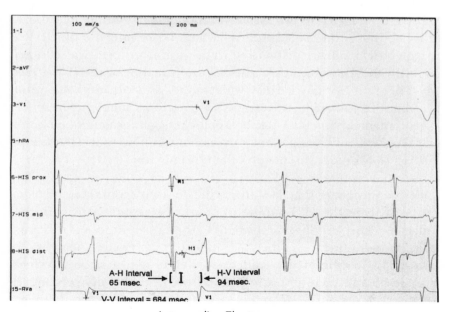

Intracardiac Electrogram

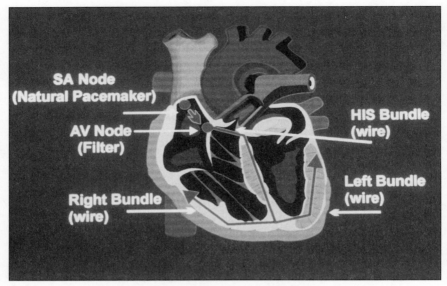

The Heart's Electrical Circuitry

minute. Much higher or much lower numbers imply possible problems with the heart's pacemaker.

2. We then measure two major components of a single heartbeat. The first is the "A-H interval," which represents the time from electrical activity of the low right atrium to electrical contact with the HIS bundle. It assesses the function of the A-V node. This number has a fairly wide range, and can depend upon many factors such as the patient's emotional state, the presence of medications such as beta blockers and calcium channel blockers, and the patient's overall autonomic tone (see Chapter 13 for more discussion of autonomic tone).

We then evaluate the "H-V interval," the time from onset of electrical activity in the HIS bundle to onset of electrical activity in the ventricles. This number is insulated from our emotional fluctuations. It does not vary as the A-H interval, but remains nearly constant and is confined to a much smaller range of normal values between 35 and 55 milliseconds. The presence of a very prolonged H-V interval (e.g., over 100 milliseconds), bodes poorly, predicting a failure of the heart's electrical wiring in the not-too-distant future.

These patients invariably receive permanent pacemakers to prevent future events such as sudden fainting spells.

In case you've fallen asleep during our discussion of basic intervals, it's time to wake up as we must now stimulate the heart. We stimulate (or pace) the heart at different frequencies and at different sites. Initially, we pace the heart from the high right atrial catheter, which you may recall lies next to our natural pacemaker, the sinus node. We pace here at different rates: 100 beats per minute, 120 beats per minute, 150 beats per minute, 200 beats per minute. We look for two things: First, how well does the sinus node respond to stress—does it take too long to recover, or does it bounce back appropriately after being bombarded by this outside energy? Second, how does the A-V node fare under these increasing rates? It is both normal and protective for the A-V node to block some impulses from reaching the ventricles at fast rates. In fact, the A-V node is truly a filter, and its function and purpose are to limit the input from reaching the ventricles, and to coordinate the input to the ventricles so they can function in synchrony, as a unit. There is an established normal range at which the A-V node should block impulses, and it is during this part of the test that either normal or abnormal A-V nodal function is again assessed.

Next, we perform programmed electrical stimulation (PES), from both the right upper and lower chambers (atrium and ventricle) of the heart. PES entails delivering eight beats at a given rate and then adding a ninth at an earlier and earlier time. A tenth and eleventh extra beat are often delivered when evaluating the ventricle. This form of stimulation stresses the heart even further, in order to try to uncover a sick heart's natural tendency to experience an abnormal rhythm. The "stress" on the heart is temporary and persists only during the moment of stimulation. It is a necessary stress, however, and can often uncover potentially life-threatening heart rhythms.

After finishing the programmed electrical stimulation, we often perform carotid sinus massage—a manual massage done to slow heart rhythms and initiate a drop in blood pressure. In most patients, the heart rate slows naturally during massage of the carotid sinus. However, if there is a pause in heartbeats of over three seconds, this may indicate that a pacemaker is required.

This is the basic electrophysiologic study that Mr. Rodriguez and many other patients undergo. It takes less than an hour to perform.

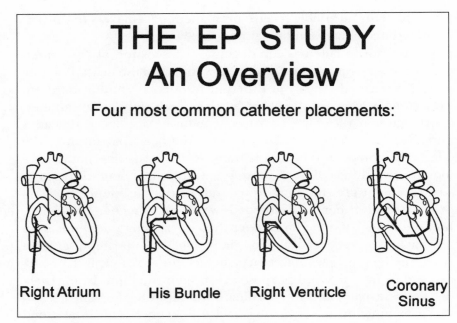

THE EP STUDY
An Overview

Four most common catheter placements:

Right Atrium   **His Bundle**   **Right Ventricle**   **Coronary Sinus**

The EP Study: An Overview

In our patient's case, a bypass tract—that extra pathway—was discovered. Energy was delivered through a catheter to burn and destroy a portion of the pathway. The circuit was thereby eliminated and Mr. Rodriguez was no longer susceptible to life-threatening heart rhythm disturbances.

Mr. Rodriguez was discharged from the hospital on the following day. He returned to soccer and roofing two days later; and now, several years since his study, he has had no recurrence of the abnormal heart rhythm. Ramon Rodriguez's story is certainly an example of one of the miracles of modern technologically based medicine.

The "Common" Faint

Imagine that it's a warm summer day and you are rushing around trying to make a noon tennis date. Because of your hurried schedule, you neglect to eat breakfast or "tank up" with plenty of fluids, and lunch is scheduled after your grueling tennis match. You reach the court exhausted but on time. Before you know it, you're in the tennis duel of the century. The perspiration is everywhere; you are running, jumping, smashing, and dripping. Your clothes are soaked and the court sizzles repeatedly with drops of your falling sweat. Between sets, you sit on the bench, towel off, look up at the beating sun, stand up, and collapse to the ground—a flaccid, pale, exhausted, wet, unconscious being. Yes, you have just fainted. Initially fearful that you've suffered a heart attack, your partner finally understands that you have fainted, and nothing more. He splashes cold water on your face and shakes you repeatedly until you stir. As you open your eyes, you're likely to feel nauseated and weak, perhaps even quite embarrassed. After resting awhile, you're able to get up, drink some nourishing liquids, eat lunch, and feel physically better (hopefully, you have not taken a hot sauna in the interim, which would certainly lead to a second faint). You go home and call your doctor. He meets you in the emergency room, where he reviews your history, does a physical examination, and takes an electrocardiogram. He determines that you are in excellent physical condition and nothing is wrong with your heart.

"Why, then, did I faint?" you may query.

"You have just experienced an episode of neurally mediated or vasovagal syncope," he responds.

Excuse me? In English, please!

I will explain the physiology of neurally mediated syncope (syncope means fainting) in the context of the test we perform to diagnose this problem—the tilt table test. Our tennis enthusiast arrives at the hospital on an outpatient basis. He is placed on a table with a footboard that can support his weight. A continuous EKG monitor and blood pressure cuff are connected and the table is tilted to a 75-degree head-upright angle. Several different protocols are used to perform this exam, some with and some without the use of adjunctive medications delivered intravenously. I usually perform this test in the "native" state, that is, without intravenous medications. The test takes 45 minutes (unless it is preempted by a fainting spell, the end point of the procedure). During this time, the patient stands still, without moving his legs. Under normal circumstances, as we walk and move about, our legs help pump blood back to our heart. During the tilt table study, the legs are immobile and so blood pools and the heart becomes less filled with blood.

This simulates the experience of our tennis player who skipped breakfast (and all the fluids that go with this meal) and then sweat profusely in the blazing sunshine. As his heart shrank in volume (what we call "empty heart syndrome"), his body tried to protect itself and maintain flow to the important organs (like the brain). To increase blood circulation, his heart beat faster and more forcefully. This is all that occurs in most people. But in our patient and others prone to "neurally mediated syncope," something goes amiss. As the heart pounds away, receptors become activated in the undersurface of the heart muscle. These receptors send a message to the brain, telling it that the heart is doing too much work. Trying to protect the heart, the brain then delivers a command to the body for the heart to slow down and the arteries to dilate (expand). As the heart slows and the blood vessels dilate, blood pressure falls. This results in a decrease in blood flow to those important organs (like the brain). The next thing that drops is the patient—right to the ground.

This describes the physiology of the most common type of faint, as occurs when having blood drawn (as my wife often does), watching an upsetting movie, standing for hours in a long line, coming out of a hot tub, or playing tennis in the hot sun. Although neurally mediated syncope is benign, it can occur frequently enough to be problematic for some people. Luckily, there are various medications that can effectively block the physiologic cycle just described. For example, beta blockers—medicines such as atenolol, propranolol, and metoprolol—blunt the increase in heart rate and force of muscle contractility. Because heart rate and force of contractility cannot increase too greatly, the receptors in the heart are never activated. Thus, the brain is not alerted to a possible problem with the heart, and so, does not initiate the events that would ultimately lead to a faint. Other medicines, like Florinef, increase the blood volume as an attempt to prevent the heart from ever achieving that "empty" state.

The problem with medicines, as always, is their potential side effects. The beta blockers can make people feel sluggish and diminish their sexual capacities, while Florinef can make patients' legs swell and cause hypertension. Some patients, of course, require medications, so physicians must evaluate the pros and cons of drug therapy on an individual basis. The tennis player just described does not require an electrophysiologic study, and in fact, if his faint is an isolated event, he probably does not even need a tilt table test. He should be cautioned to avoid circumstances that may provoke fainting. He should eat regularly, consume ample fluids, and avoid exercising in excessive heat. He should not drink alcohol prior to performing significant physical activity, and he should avoid standing still for prolonged periods of time. Additionally, hot showers and saunas are generally off limits.

Making these minor lifestyle adjustments may be enough to spare many patients any further fainting spells. If, however, a person were to experience recurrent fainting from neurally mediated syncope, then a tilt table could be used to guide therapy. Medications will be adjusted to ensure that the patient does not faint during the tilt. When this is accomplished, the patient's prognosis is excellent, and he or she can feel reassured that recurrent episodes of fainting will not be in his or her future.

In conclusion, remember this: While electrical problems with the heart can be very complex and frightening, they often are manageable with appropriate reassurance and guidance. This is an area in cardiology which is evolving at an extraordinarily rapid rate. With patients unfortunate enough to have malignant or potentially lethal forms of rhythm disturbances, there are now curative or preventive therapies, which can prolong life in ways that were never possible before.

If you're curious and want to learn more about a variety of electrophysiologic ailments, you can turn to the Appendix, where they are described in detail.

If Chicken Soup Is Penicillin, Then What Is This I'm Eating?

I was raised on a "balanced diet." Meat, potatoes, vegetables, milk, and cookies represented my typical dinner. The concept of "balance," however, has taken tortuous twists and turns over the last several decades. The nutritional playing field has become so muddied that it often seems impossible to be sure that you are traveling in the right direction. Butter is bad, so margarine is introduced. Then margarine is bad, and butter is redeemed. Meat is bad; vegetarianism is good. Then Dr. Robert Atkins comes along and tells us to toss our vegetables in the garbage and turn our attention to bacon, eggs, and hot dogs. While Dr. Atkins lavishes lumps of lard upon us, Dr. Dean Ornish—the first medical doctor to demonstrate that it's possible to reverse heart disease without invasive treatments such as bypass surgery—advises only a modicum of fats for heart health. Meanwhile, Dr. D'Adamo, a naturopath, instructs us to have our blood type assessed prior to formulating an appropriate nutritional regimen.

From Atkins to vegetarianism, the gamut of dietary choices is rife with possibilities. What are we supposed to do to maintain health benefits while achieving slender forms? Is there a perfect diet that suits all of us, or does each of us have to find his or her own way among the many possibilities?

In this chapter, I will explore several of the diets that are currently *en vogue*. It is my hope, of course, that by chapter's end, you will have a sense of which diet may be best for you. As a diet must be tailored to an individual, you may want a nutritionist to assist you in your search.

Before discussing the various dietary options now available to us, however, we should examine the three basic components of all food substances—what nutritionists call "the macromolecules"—carbohydrates, proteins, and fats.

Carbohydrates

Scientifically speaking, carbohydrates represent a class of compounds in the form $Cn(H_2O)n$. This of, course, means very little to most people. But translated into everyday language, carbohydrates are compounds made up of the sugars and starches.

Carbohydrates are further subdivided into simple and complex. Simple carbohydrates have between one and ten saccharides units (i.e., sugar/starch units) strung together, while complex carbohydrates are *poly*saccharides, having many simple carbohydrates linked together, creating a more complex structure.

Most carbohydrate-containing foods actually represent a combination of both simple and complex forms. The most common *mono*saccharides—the simplest of the simple carbohydrates—are glucose, fructose, and galactose. These three compounds are the building blocks of the more complex carbohydrates.

Glucose, our body's most important fuel, is the "giant" of the monosaccharides. All carbohydrates consumed ultimately end up as glucose, which we then use in one of three ways. It can be immediately metabolized to meet the body's current energy demands, it can be stored in the liver and muscle as glycogen, or it can be converted to fat and stored as adipose tissue—body fat.

Fructose, the sweetest of the simple sugars, is found mostly in fruits and, to a lesser degree, in vegetables which are nutrient-dense, high-fiber foods. Consuming fructose may effect a smaller rise in blood glucose levels than consuming equivalent amounts of sucrose and starchy carbohydrates. As you will discover, a smaller rise in glucose translates into a smaller rise in insulin, resulting eventually in a decrease in the production of fat. Do not feel, however, that this gives you carte blanche to consume fruits indiscriminately. In my clinical experience, the high sugar content of a diet based on fruit often leads to unwanted weight gain.

Other monosaccharides which also yield more blunted rises in the blood (serum) glucose levels are the "sugar alcohols": sorbitol, mannitol, and xylitol, which are added to some foods but not usually found in nature.

For their part, the disaccharides—two monosaccharides joined together—comprise another group of simple sugars. Sucrose, the most well known of the disaccharides (the common form of table sugar), is a combination of glucose and fructose. Lactose, the combination of glucose and galactose, is the sugar that lends milk its sweetness.

When three to ten monosaccharide units are linked, an *oligo*saccharide—another simple sugar—results. Stachyose and raffinose, the most commonly occurring oligosaccharides, are found in small amounts in legumes and lentils.

*Poly*saccharides, or starches, are sugars composed of more than ten monosaccharide units, and include potatoes, pasta, and bread. It's a common misconception that these foods are simple carbohydrates; they are actually complex carbohydrates. Just because they are "complex" carbohydrates, however, does not imply that they are good for you.

Another common misconception is that complex carbohydrates are good. In fact, it is the high fiber content of foods containing complex carbohydrates that can endow them with health benefits. Complex carbohydrates not high in fiber—like pasta, bread, and potatoes—also fail to confer the same health benefits as complex carbohydrates that are high in fiber, like vegetables and beans.

Thus, if you eat bread, eat whole grain, unprocessed bread, not white bread, which has very little food value. The same goes for pasta, making whole wheat pasta a must. Of course, the most healthful grains are the ones you must cook for 20–30 minutes, like oats or brown rice. As unprocessed foods, they contain all the nutritive value destroyed during the processing that creates white flour or rice.

Now fiber, or roughage, is an indigestible form of carbohydrates. Although there are many ways that fiber contributes health benefits, its capacity to decrease the overall speed of carbohydrate absorption by the intestinal tract is first on the list. By lowering the rate of absorption of carbohydrates, a more tempered rise in glucose—and thus insulin—occurs, and so less carbohydrate is converted to unwanted fat.

Fiber can be further subdivided into soluble and insoluble groups. This terminology, perhaps not the most accurate, at least enables us to segregate fibers into meaningful categories with regard to their ability to lower or not lower cholesterol.

The *soluble* fibers such as guar gum, psyllium, and pectin are excellent additions to our cholesterol-lowering armamentarium. They have the added benefit of decreasing stool transit time, thus helping to eliminate constipation, diverticular disease, and other intestinal abnormalities.

The *insoluble* fibers, like wheat bran, do not have the capability of lowering cholesterol levels to any significant degree, but they do benefit bowel function.

Both soluble and insoluble fibers should be plentiful in our diets; yet they represent foods most commonly absent in the American meal plan. Foods containing large amounts of excellent forms of fiber—vegetables and legumes—have been shown, in numerous studies, to promote such health benefits as lowering blood pressure, cholesterol and glucose levels, and decreasing the incidence of cardiovascular disease.

Fat

Over the past decade or so, fats have been stigmatized. While it is true that consuming an overabundance of certain fats will lead to cardiovascular and other diseases, these compounds should not be blindly and uniformly eliminated from our diets. Fats are required as building blocks of every cell in our bodies. They are also essential in the proper development of hormones and neural structures. We cannot live without fat.

Of the fats we consume, 99 percent are triglycerides, unions of a single glycerol structure and three fatty acids. Most triglycerides are long-chained, composed of 12–30 carbon atoms with their attached hydrogen and oxygen molecules. Fats are defined as being either fully saturated, *mono*unsaturated, or *poly*unsaturated.

These distinctions between the types of fats are based on their chemical structures. The saturated fats contain no double bonds, while the monounsaturated fats contain a single double bond, and the polyunsaturated fats contain two or more double bonds.

In your reading, you may have observed that a number is often attached to the name of various fatty acids; for example, omega-3, omega-6, and omega-9 fatty acids. This number actually refers to the position of the first double bond. The omega-3 fatty acids EPA and DHA, for instance, have their first double bond at the third position. The omega-9 fatty acid—oleic acid, a major component of olive and canola oils—has its first and only double bond at the ninth position. Oleic acid is thus a *mono*unsaturated fatty acid.

Food sources usually represent a conglomeration of various fats; while one type of fat may predominate, a variety of fats is usually present. Certainly, the consumption of saturated fats, such as butter and palm and coconut oil, predisposes patients to developing high cholesterol and coronary artery disease. These saturated fats, you will note, are solid at room temperature. The monounsaturated fats, such as oleic acid, are present in high quantities in olive and canola oil and many nuts and seeds. These fats, which are liquid at room temperature, have a protective and beneficial effect on cholesterol, lowering triglycerides, LDL, and total cholesterol levels. The polyunsaturated fatty acids, containing two or more "double bonds," are present in high quantities in vegetable oils such as soybean oil. These, too, are liquid at room temperature. Although they lack the same cardiovascular benefits as the monounsaturated fatty acids, they are certainly not so bad as the saturated fatty acids. In fact, two polyunsaturated fatty acids, linolenic (omega-3) and linoleic (omega-6), are "essential," meaning our bodies are incapable of producing them. We must, therefore, consume them in our diet.

We are learning as well that the limited consumption of these essential fatty acids in the typical American diet has led to numerous health problems. Of course, the best way to increase linolenic acid and other omega-3 fatty acids such as DHA and EPA is by eating large quantities of marine fish, walnuts, and flaxseed oil. However, this is often impractical, and so omega-3 fatty acid supplements should be taken to ensure adequate dietary intake.

Deserving of special attention are the trans-fatty acids. It's through the hydrogenation of *liquid* oils that trans-fatty acids are made, specifically to remain *solid* at room temperature as margarine does. Trans-fatty acids, however, are unnatural and potentially harmful substances. Simply put, the trans-fatty acids take on characteristics even worse than those of the saturated fatty acids, increasing total cholesterol and LDL while lowering HDL, the heart-protective cholesterol. Fried foods, snack foods, commercially baked foods, margarine, and various commercial salad dressings (such as ranch dressing) all contain high quantities of trans-fatty acids.

Because trans-fatty acids have been linked to cancers, increased LDL cholesterol, and decreased HDL cholesterol, avoid them as much as you can! At the same time, remember that it is not the general category of "fats" that is the enemy, but the subsets of fats, such as the saturated and trans-fatty acids, which cause us so many problems. In addition, it is not just the fats that make people fat; carbohydrates and excess quantities of food can promote obesity as well.

TABLE 21
Dr. Baum's List of Desirable Foods for
Cardiovascular Health

I recommend a diet replete with these foods because they are high in vitamins, minerals, phytonutrients, and fiber, and have a low glycemic index (i.e., are absorbed slowly).

Nonstarchy, High-Fiber Vegetables	Grains and Starchy Vegetables
onions	oatmeal/bran
broccoli	brown rice
peppers (all varieties)	wheat germ
tomato	sweet potato
kale	barley
celery	sprouted grain breads
spinach	
asparagus	
romaine lettuce	
artichoke	

Beans and Legumes	Protein Sources
All beans are desirable, because of their high-fiber content, but some are higher in calcium and magnesium than others, and they are ranked as follows:	salmon
	tuna
	herring
	sardines (with bones)
	tofu/tempeh (soy protein)
soybeans	shrimp
white beans	turkey breast
navy beans	white meat chicken (no skin)
black beans	egg
red beans	
lima beans	
black-eyed peas	
chickpeas	

TABLE 21 (Continued)
Dr. Baum's List of Desirable Foods for
Cardiovascular Health

Nuts, Seeds, and Fat	Fruits
flaxseed oil (never heat this oil)	grapefruit
grape seed oil	orange
canola oil	kiwi
olive oil	strawberries
almonds	cantaloupe
walnuts	banana (underripe)
avocado	grapes
	apricots
	apple

Protein

Protein, the third and final macromolecule that constitutes what we eat, is an immensely important contributor to energy and growth. Amino acids are the building blocks of all proteins. Twenty amino acids occur naturally and nine are "essential"—they are required components of our diets, as they cannot be manufactured within our bodies, including: histidine, isoleucine, leucine, lysine, methionine, phenylalanine, threonine, tryptophan, and valine. We can produce the other eleven amino acids through our body's metabolic machinery; thus their absence will not necessarily result in disease.

In evaluating the protein present in foods, scientists can establish "biological values"—a measure of which proteins our bodies can utilize for growth or maintenance of normal functions. High-biological-value proteins are more "complete" than low-biological proteins, as they contain all the essential amino acids. The protein in eggs, meat, fish, and milk have a very high biological value, whereas nuts, seeds, and vegetables do not contain all the essential amino acids and hence have a lower biological value.

While carbohydrates and fats are stored by the body, proteins and amino acids are not. Instead, they exist in a continuous cycle of creation and degradation. In other words, proteins are constantly being "turned over" in our bodies. The resultant amino acids are shifted and recycled, forming new and different protein structures.

Protein breakdown results in the creation of nitrogen, which has many ways of leaving our bodies—through the urine, stool, sweat, and even through our skin, hair, and nails. To be certain that we're in good protein balance though, we must all consume more protein than we eliminate. For the average person, it's recommended that he or she consume approximately 0.8 gram of protein per kilogram of body weight. Thus, a 100-kilogram man should eat approximately 80 grams of protein from a combination of sources every day. Physically active individuals, like weight lifters, should probably maintain a daily protein consumption of between 1 and 1.2 grams per kilogram of body weight.

The energy value of proteins and carbohydrates is equivalent; both supply approximately 4 calories per gram. Fat, on the other hand, is much more caloric, containing 9 calories per gram. Fat is thus the most efficient means of *storing* energy, enabling us to squeeze larger energy stores into a smaller space. When we eat fat, however, we are consuming far more calories per serving than when we eat protein or carbohydrate; thus, fats are more "fattening" than protein or carbohydrates.

What's for Dinner?

A multitude of popular diets baffle me when I scan the shelves of my local bookstores. Like most Americans, my wife and I have tried to find our way through such dietary possibilities, and as I describe some of the decisions we've made, I'll detail today's more popular diets.

My wife has suffered from weight fluctuations throughout her life. Although she is not obese, she occasionally puts on enough weight to make herself feel both uncomfortable and distressed. She, like a multitude of other women, has tried countless popular diets. On occasion, these diets were transiently successful. She would lose weight, find the diet impossible to maintain, and then regain whatever weight she had lost. Recently, however, she read a book by Philip Lipetz, Ph.D., called *Naturally Slim and Powerful*. The emphasis of his diet is to enhance serotonin levels, a fascinating and intelligent approach to weight loss in women.

Dr. Lipetz's basic premise is that men and women are different. As Lipetz notes, women normally have much higher brain levels of serotonin than do men. This, perhaps, explains some of the "superior" mental attributes many women possess. Additionally, serotonin influences behaviors such as sexuality, appetite, mood, and stress response, thus greatly influencing the maintenance of a woman's emotional balance and stability. When a woman's serotonin levels fall, she may gain weight, become depressed or stressed, experience worsening premenstrual syndrome, have a decreased libido, experience increased food cravings, and become irritable. For women (and the men who love them), this is a bad thing. Dr. Lipetz points out that most modern diets tend to *decrease* the serotonin levels in women within a matter of just three weeks.

Some diets increase insulin levels and, therefore, increase serotonin levels, but only briefly. This can result in a vicious cycle in which the dieter begins to crave carbohydrates. Carbohydrates can increase insulin, which then increases tryptophan, which in turn augments serotonin levels. Unfortunately, this serotonin rise is brief, lasting only about six hours, and subsequently dropping precipitously to very low levels. The dieter must then consume more carbohydrates, obviating the diet and allowing for an increase in fat creation and weight gain. Carbohydrates, in this regard, are not so different from other "drugs" which tend to increase serotonin levels—like tobacco and alcohol.

In his book, Dr. Lipetz establishes a dietary regimen for women which increases and maintains high serotonin levels. (Antidepressants such as Prozac also raise serotonin levels, but it's far superior for most people, of course, to attempt to increase their amounts of this neurotransmitter with a natural method like diet.) Not only is the quality of one's food important, but also the timing of what and when to eat, at least to maintain high serotonin levels. For example, Dr. Lipetz states that proteins should be eaten separately from serotonin-raising foods, and should also be eliminated from a typical breakfast. When my wife "lived" this diet, she was amazed at not only how simple but also at how effective it was at reducing her weight and improving her mood. She has truly thrived on Dr. Lipetz's dietary recommendations. Although this is perhaps not one of the most popular of all diets, it is, I feel, one of the most scientifically sound, especially in relation to the unique needs of women.

A personalized version of the Lipetz diet that my wife now utilizes consists of the following: Her morning meal is high in complex carbohydrates. It is a substantial meal with limited, if any, protein. A typical breakfast includes slow-cooked oatmeal with applesauce and cinnamon instead of milk and brown sugar, because there is too much protein in the milk. The reason to avoid protein in the morning is that high dietary intake of protein limits the amount of tryptophan that can be used by the brain and converted into serotonin. Therefore, serotonin levels will be lower in patients eating a high-protein diet. Again, the thrust of this diet is to enable the body to increase the natural production of serotonin. High serotonin levels will help prevent mood swings and carbohydrate cravings.

Another typical breakfast might include grapefruit and a baked sweet potato. Most traditional (and commercial) breakfast cereals are too high in sugar and promote fat production. Neither is yogurt a good choice for breakfast, again because it has a fairly high protein content that will interfere with serotonin production. If you eat a banana for breakfast, it should be underripe as opposed to overripe, because underripe fruit contains less sugar.

Lunch should be eaten rather late in the day, and consist of complex carbohydrates such as brown rice (which is vastly superior to white rice) with a modicum of protein. The preferable protein source in this diet is legumes. A typical meal includes a salad with chickpeas and a variety of vegetables. Chicken or fish, in small portions, is acceptable at lunch. This enables the body to digest and metabolize the protein long before the following morning's breakfast.

Dinner also consists primarily of complex carbohydrates, slow-cooked grains, and vegetables. One of my wife's favorite meals is a wintertime chili containing such delectable ingredients as butternut squash, onions, garlic, tomatoes, corn, celery, and black beans. Note that the onions and garlic add a cardiovascular benefit independent of the diet's good weight loss and mental health–promoting elements. This wintertime chili has the added benefit of being easily stored. It can be cooked in a large quantity and then reheated quickly and easily for additional meals during the week. Alternatively, my wife frequently eats a delicious assortment of brown rice, vegetables, and beans. Chickpeas and other beans are great additives to lunch and dinner recipes. For women in search of a scientifically sound, gender-specific method for weight reduction and mood enhancement, this diet represents an excellent choice.

Peter J. D'Adamo, N.D., has also written a fascinating and provocative book, *Eat Right for Your Type,* which addresses dietary recommendations in the context of blood types. For D'Adamo, human beings' blood types evolved in association with environmental influences such as changing dietary habits. Dr. D'Adamo refers to the fact that Cro-Magnon man, living 40,000 years ago, carried only Type O blood within his veins. During his reign, he was at the top of the food chain, being a worthy adversary to all forms of prey—in other words, a dominant meat eater. His great success at hunting led to a huge population expansion, ultimately causing him to seek out new territories for acquisition of adequate food. This stimulated his migration from Africa through Europe and much of Asia.

As Dr. D'Adamo relates it, by 10,000 B.C., people existed on every single land mass in the world, with the exception of Antarctica. During the Neolithic period, or the "New Stone Age" approximately 15,000 years ago, both farming and animal husbandry were born. It is during this era that Type A blood emerged, and along with it appeared certain digestive tract and immune system alterations. These other changes allowed people to achieve better absorption of grains, which had previously been absent from their diets. Blood Type B evolved around 10,000 years ago in the Himalayan highlands currently representing Pakistan and India. Dr. D'Adamo claims that this change in blood type resulted not from dietary influences, as in type A, but rather from climatic changes. The diet of these people, however, was transformed as well, with an increased consumption of meat and cultured dairy products.

It is interesting and somewhat confusing to note that many modern-day Jews have Type B blood, *regardless* of their national origin. Scientists who study population genetics usually attribute this to what is called the "founder effect"—that is, that most Jews living today descended originally from a very small number of founders. Other groups with an extremely high prevalence of Type B blood include Japanese, Chinese, and Indians.

Type AB blood is mankind's most recent evolutionary blood type metamorphosis, emerging only about 1,000 years age. People with type AB are purportedly blessed with fewer allergies and autoimmune disorders, but some cancers have been found to be more prevalent in those bearing this blood.

The connection between blood types and food recommendations is derived from the diverse interaction of lectins—proteins in all foods—with blood cells of different types. Lectins give foods "gluelike" properties, such that when ingested in the "wrong" individual, they will cause a clumping of blood cells. For example, milk is similar to Type B blood, and thus when a Type A individual consumes it, he or she will experience an agglutination (clumping) of blood. Obviously, this agglutination is on a small scale and should have little or no serious aftereffects.

Of all the lectins consumed, 95 percent are filtered out and never enter our bloodstream. The remaining 5 percent, however, represent the potential "clumpers" of our blood supply, according to Dr. D'Adamo.

When I first heard of Dr. D'Adamo's diet, I, like many others, took it as another wacky, even ridiculous plan. After reading his book, however, I discovered that some of his suggestions have a reasonably sound scientific base. So it is not unreasonable to give his dietary recommendations a try. You really have nothing to lose—and perhaps a great deal to gain. Unfortunately, having had no personal experience with this diet, I cannot share any anecdotal reports about it with you.

Balance, although desirable in all aspects of life, is often not achieved with some of the more popular dietary recommendations. The Atkins diet is the worst culprit here, one of the least well balanced of all popular diets. Dr. Atkins wisely states that many obese people are "carbohydrate sensitive," and even carbohydrate addicted. He uses this truth, however, to justify a diet that, although solving the problem of carbohydrate addiction, results in a very unhealthy existence. When patients are carbohydrate sensitive, they are resistant to their own insulin. Thus, they require excessive levels of insulin to achieve the same physiological result that ordinarily would occur with normal insulin levels. This "hyperinsulinemia" results in an augmentation of glucose's undesired conversion to fat, ultimately leading to weight gain. A vicious cycle ensues in which patients consume more and more carbohydrates, raising their insulin levels ever higher and causing the formation of more and more fat.

To break this cycle, Dr. Atkins advocates the use of a diet which shuns carbohydrates, and comprises only proteins and fatty foods. This "unnatural" diet results in a state of ketosis, during which time fat is burned as an energy source. Although Dr. Atkins poetically and humorously describes ketosis as "one of life's charmed gifts . . . as delightful as sex and sunshine with fewer drawbacks than either of them," what he neglects to share with the reader is that this diet can be dangerous. Bad breath, constipation, dehydration, loss of muscle mass, osteoporosis, and depleted glycogen stores are just a few of the potential consequences of this diet.

Although patients often justify the Atkins diet by bragging about an increase in their HDLs (the protective component of cholesterol), what they fail to understand is that this represents an adaptive and transient response. It occurs only in the body's efforts to transport the excess fat floating in the bloodstream that results from this unbalanced diet. The Atkins diet demands the consumption of high quantities of animal protein laden with saturated fats, which numerous studies have shown can lead to the development of subsequent heart disease, cancers, and osteoporosis. His diet also claims that wonderful foods like fruits and complex carbohydrates are "bad." To so classify foods that have been documented by numerous studies as health-promoting—associated with lower risks of high blood pressure, heart disease, diabetes, and cancers—is, I feel, a terrible misrepresentation.

Sure, people lose weight with the Atkins diet, but at what price? The Atkins diet is the adult equivalent of telling children that they can solve their dietary problems by entering any candy store and eating whatever they desire. People want to be told that eating bacon and eggs, roast beef, hot dogs, and hamburgers is good for them. It isn't. My recommendation is to stay away from the Atkins diet unless a nutritionist or physician finds that this is the only method whereby weight loss *induction* can occur. If this is the case, then a modified Atkins diet—utilizing lean proteins and monounsaturated fatty acids—can be followed. As far as the permanent diet goes, avoid it. If it helps you to begin to lose weight, and this is necessary for your long-term health, fine. But staying on the Atkins diet for the rest of your life is, in my opinion, a very unhealthful decision to make.

Ornish and Pritikin (first Nathan Pritikin and now Robert Pritikin) have developed diets that are nearly the antitheses of the Atkins diet. Both Pritikin and Ornish require very high carbohydrate intake, with carbohydrates representing approximately 75 percent of total calories. Compare this to the less than 5 percent of total calories that carbohydrates represent in the Atkins diet. Protein intake is only about 15 percent in both Pritikin and Ornish, whereas fat is less than or equal to 10 percent of total caloric intake. While the content of fiber is high in both Ornish and Pritikin, it is extremely low, if not negligible, in the Atkins diet. Fiber, as you know, has numerous health-promoting benefits.

If I were to choose between Pritikin or Ornish, and the Atkins diet, there is no question that I would fall on the side of Pritikin and Ornish. My problem with both of these diets, however, is their limitation of fat and protein intake. (They are also very difficult diets to follow on a long-term basis.) Fats, as you now know, are not all bad. In fact, some are essential for life. Unfortunately, neither Ornish nor Pritikin does justice to the importance of fats. I agree that the saturated fats are bad, but to brand all polyunsaturated and monounsaturated fats as bad is clearly wrong.

Consider, for example, the Cretan or Mediterranean diet. In this diet, carbohydrates represent over 50 percent of calories; proteins are unspecified and fat is 25–35 percent of total caloric intake. Most of the "Mediterranean" fats, however, are unsaturated, with saturated fats representing less than 7 percent of total caloric intake. This Cretan, or Mediterranean, diet has been shown to decrease the risk of cardiovascular disease (and may protect against cancer and other diseases, as well). In fact, a recent study demonstrated that Cretan men experience the lowest incidence of heart disease of all cultures examined. These people consume fish, vegetables and olive oil, and use meat sparingly, as an additive to a meal rather than as the focus of a meal. They do not consume anything even vaguely resembling the vegetarian diet recommended by Pritikin and Ornish. In favor of Ornish, however, I must admit that he did demonstrate mild coronary artery disease regression in a subgroup of patients consuming his diet while simultaneously meditating and exercising vigorously. While it is thus not clear that the diet alone was the key to the cardiovascular success in his study—nearly equal emphasis was placed on exercise and meditation—we cannot dismiss its potential importance.

I think the Cretan diet is excellent, and it is clearly associated with a low incidence of coronary artery disease. Nevertheless, I prefer the Lipetz diet for women, for all the reasons stated above, and the Zone diet for men, which we will consider now.

Barry Sears, Ph.D., created the Zone diet. Without a doubt, it is my favorite popular diet for men. I say this from experience, as I have "lived" the Zone diet. I feel my best when I follow a Zone diet. My weight is controlled, I have less hunger, and overall, I just feel better.

The Zone diet is one of the most well balanced of all popular programs. It is composed of 40 percent carbohydrates, 30 percent protein, and 30 percent fat. Consuming saturated fats is discouraged, whereas consumption of monounsaturated and polyunsaturated fats is encouraged. It is advised that cholesterol intake remain under 300 mg a day.

Dr. Sears uses the same facts about hyperinsulinemia as Dr. Atkins to create a substantially different diet. Dr. Sears's diet is heart-friendly, whereas Dr. Atkins's is not. In the Zone diet, it is not just the total quantities of carbohydrate, protein, and fat that are stressed, it is also the *balance* of each of these macromolecules in every meal that contributes to this diet's success. Dr. Sears states that each meal should balance protein, carbohydrate, and fat in order to help decrease the rate of entry of carbohydrates into the bloodstream. As you already know, a slower absorption of carbohydrates will blunt the insulin response and thus diminish fat production.

Dr. Sears, like several other nutritional advisors, uses the "glycemic index" as a guide to understanding carbohydrate absorption. Foods with "high" indices are absorbed rapidly and thus are "bad." Foods with low glycemic indices are absorbed slowly and thus are "good." Because of their high glycemic index, refined carbohydrates such as flour and starches are eliminated from the Zone diet. Beans, fruits, and fibrous vegetables with low glycemic indices are strongly favored. The diet's emphasis is thus on lean protein sources, mono-unsaturated fats, and low glycemic carbohydrates.

Dr. Sears pays special attention to the production of eicosanoids, hormone-like substances that we create from the essential fatty acids, and their role in preventing or promoting disease. He points out that high levels of insulin lead not only to weight gain but also can cause the production of the "bad" eicosanoids such as arachidonic acid (which, by the way, is replete in animal fat, à la Atkins). These substances can increase blood pressure, constrict our vessels, and cause platelets to aggregate and blood to clot. Hardening of the arteries (atherosclerosis) may be promoted by arachidonic acid. Thus, by blunting the insulin response, the level of bad eicosanoids is diminished and the development of diseases may be deterred.

On both a scientific and a personal basis, I love the Zone diet for men. On the other hand, I must caution women, as I have not seen great success when women attempt to adhere to its recommendations. My wife, for example, did very poorly on the Zone diet; she lost no weight and felt no better. When she switched to the diet recommended by Dr. Lipetz, her mood improved, her weight decreased, and her stamina increased. Not intending to beat a dead horse, I will reiterate that diets must be individualized. The Zone diet and serotonin-enhancing diets can be backbones for slightly altered but individually more acceptable dietary regimens. I am also convinced that nutritional guidance and counseling is paramount when attempting to find a diet that suits you best.

The macrobiotic diet represents another extreme example of eating. When on a macrobiotic diet, we generally consume greater than 50 percent of our food in the form of brown rice. The remainder of the daily intake is represented by foods such as sea vegetables, fruits, vegetables, nuts, and seeds. As meat and fish are absent, the diet provides very low levels of fat and protein. Some of the essential fatty acids, however, are found in the seeds and nuts consumed by patients on the macrobiotic regimen. Although protein is present in numerous vegetables, it is generally not the same quality—i.e., it is of lower biological value than the protein found in meat and fish. To that end, I understand the macrobiotic diet as unnatural and I usually do not recommend its use on a long-term basis.

As a "jump-start" mechanism, the cabbage soup diet bears mentioning as well. That this is a *temporary* diet is sometimes forgotten, but that is its intention. In fact, it should be used for only three to seven days as a means of beginning more permanent dietary changes. Should you be so interested, I refer you to Margaret Danbrot's book, *The New Cabbage Soup Diet.* But remember: Americans, now as then, are attracted to the quick fix. Whether in relation to looks (as with liposuction and breast enlargement) or with diets (as with the cabbage soup diet), we are drawn to quick and easy solutions. The quick way, however, is not necessarily the best way. I, for one, would rather have my patients avoid diets that function as "jump starts" altogether. Be that as it may, I do understand that some people cannot find the motivation to diet unless they see rapid results. For such people, the cabbage soup diet is a reasonable approach. Just as reasonable, though, is the vegetable juice fast. In either case, I always advise my patients to diet under the strict supervision of a nutritionist or a physician when embarking on any intense and dramatic dietary regimen.

Since we have discussed many of the different ways to consume food, let's also discuss the notion of not eating—or, fasting. Fasting has recently become a more popular means of cleansing the body of toxins, including pollutants and chemicals, that have accumulated over the years. James F. Balsch, M.D., and Phyllis A. Balsch, C.N.C., in their book *Prescription for Nutritional Healing* describe a quite reasonable fasting technique. They suggest that for two days prior to fasting, people eat only raw vegetables and fruits. Subsequently, during the three- to ten-day fast, the Balschs recommend that people consume at least eight 8-ounce glasses of distilled water, vegetable juices, and up to two cups of herbal tea a day. Balsch and Balsch claim that by completing this type of fast a variety of illnesses can be warded off and energy restored to more youthful levels. They also warn that during the fast, one may suffer from a variety of ailments such as body odor, fatigue, headaches, and irritability. As I have not yet fasted (other than during Yom Kippur, for religious reasons), I cannot comment on the veracity of their assertions. I do, however, know many people who have undergone fasts and attest to their beneficial effects. Therefore, I believe that fasting probably does promote significant overall health benefits and could be incorporated into all of our annual regimens. While fasting, however, I would recommend that patients be under the strict supervision of their physicians.

Before departing this chapter, I feel compelled to discuss a very sensitive subject in a world of nutrition: the egg. A longtime breakfast favorite of the American household, the egg has taken quite a beating over the past ten to twenty years. With the knowledge of cholesterol's importance in the genesis of coronary artery disease came the condemnation of the egg, one of the most significant sources of dietary cholesterol, containing 215 mg of cholesterol per egg.

The egg's bad reputation, however, is only partially justified. Sure, eggs contain high quantities of cholesterol, but cholesterol consumption has only a minimal impact on blood cholesterol levels (saturated fat consumption is much more consequential). For example, reducing dietary cholesterol by 33 percent will result in only a 1–2 percent fall in blood cholesterol levels. An exception to this rests in patients with combined hyperlipidemia (i.e., with elevated cholesterol *and* triglyceride levels), where cholesterol consumption has been shown to have a much greater impact on blood cholesterol levels. Besides the egg's cholesterol content, its other negative characteristic includes a high content of arachidonic acid, the precursor of undesirable prostaglandins. Limiting egg consumption, however, is neither the only way nor the best way to diminish your intake of arachidonic acid. For instance, decreasing red meat consumption and supplementing one's diet with the omega-3 fatty acids will have a greater impact on creating the "good" prostaglandins (naturally made hormones we require for good health) while simultaneously limiting the "bad" prostaglandins.

Do eggs have positive attributes? It turns out that eggs are one of nature's most nutritious foods, providing the highest quality protein, numerous vitamins, trace minerals, and iron. In fact, a single egg has over 6 grams of protein, 60 percent of it within the egg white and 40 percent in the egg yolk. Not only are eggs high-protein foods, but they are also high-*quality* protein foods, containing all of the essential amino acids in proper proportion for excellent human nutrition. Eggs are also one of the few food sources that contain vitamin D. Yes, eggs are not all bad. And if you consume two or three whole eggs per week, I would not advise you to do otherwise. In fact, it's probably even *beneficial* to consume two or three eggs a week.

While we're talking about eggs, what about coffee? The impact of caffeine consumption has been a point of considerable controversy in cardiovascular health. Caffeine will clearly elevate both blood pressure and heart rate when consumed sporadically and copiously. In patients who drink *moderate* amounts of coffee on a *regular* basis, the cardiovascular effects are blunted. It is standard medical practice, however, to limit coffee consumption in all patients with significant high blood pressure or rapid heart rhythms (tachycardias). It is also important not to forget that we are more than just our hearts; coffee consumption has also been linnked in some studies to a variety of cancers. Thus, I generally advise my patients to limit their intake of coffee to one or two cups per day. I feel that this is a safe enough quantity to limit the likelihood of promoting heart disease or cancer while still allowing us to savor this great legal stimulant.

I hope I have clarified some of the salient issues surrounding dietary recommendations. My belief is that there is no single diet that fits everyone. Each of us is an individual, different and distinct from each other. Yet, as human beings, we are all imbued with the same basic rules of nature. Just as each of us has a unique set of fingerprints on a common five-fingered hand, so it is with diets. Diets should be seen as the five-fingered skeleton on which to place a more detailed and individualized imprint. When going on a diet, start with one that is balanced. Do not be lured by the sex appeal of the more exotic and outlandish diets. Consult a nutritionist. You will be investing much effort in your new dietary regimen, and to have the advice of an expert, although slightly more time-consuming and expensive than doing it on your own, will definitely be worthwhile in the long run.

Please also understand that eating disorders (i.e., emotional eating) are endemic in our time. We must often spend months—even years—of intensive introspection, at times with the help of professional counselors, to get to the bottom of these problems. Whatever the costs, time, and effort, conquering this affliction is a worthy undertaking. After all, we owe it to ourselves to make the greatest possible efforts to achieve optimal health.

Finally, I wish you all good eating in good health.

TABLE 22
Food Sources of Important Nutrients

Nutrient	Food Source
Beta-carotene	Legumes, carrots, dark leafy greens, apricots, sweet potatoes
Vitamin B$_1$ (thiamin)	Soybeans, sunflower and sesame seeds, rice bran, oatmeal, organ meats
Vitamin B$_2$ (riboflavin)	Broccoli, dark leafy greens, milk, yogurt, cottage cheese
Vitamin B$_3$ (niacin)	Organ meats, eggs, tofu, peanuts, peas
Folic acid	Broccoli, dark leafy greens, orange juice, liver, eggs
Vitamin B$_5$ (pantothenic acid)	Broccoli, salmon, eggs, turkey, chicken, royal bee jelly
Vitamin B$_6$ (pyroxidine)	Oatmeal, sunflower seeds, halibut, soybeans, bananas, avocados, animal protein
Vitamin B$_{12}$	Animal protein, oysters, tuna, cottage cheese
Biotin	Oat bran, mushrooms, pecans, almonds

TABLE 22 (Continued)
Food Sources of Important Nutrients

Nutrient	Food Source
Vitamin C	Citrus, broccoli, kiwi, red and green peppers
Vitamin D	Milk, salmon, sunshine
Vitamin E	Dark leafy greens, liver, chickpeas
Calcium	Dark leafy greens, especially kale, legumes, salmon, almonds, soybeans
Zinc	Oysters, liver, lentils, soybeans, Swiss and ricotta cheese
Manganese	Tofu, whole wheat, pineapple, chickpeas
Potassium	Bananas, flounder, yogurt, spinach, dark leafy green vegetables, legumes, wine
Magnesium	Tofu, brown rice, halibut, legumes
Copper	Sweet potatoes, tahini, oysters, legumes
Selenium	Lobster, milk, Brazil nuts
Cobalt	Animal protein
Molybdenum	Spinach, lentils, peas, cauliflower
Phosphorus	Dairy, legumes, whole grains
Chromium	Brewer's yeast, whole grains, mushrooms, nuts, wine
Iron	Liver, beef, lamb, oysters, spinach, oatmeal, sunflower seeds, cashew nuts

How the Health Food Store Can Help Your Heart

I began my foray into the field of natural medicine with the exploration of vitamins and minerals, later branching out into nutritional supplements. Being trained in traditional medicine, I believed that the answers to all medical questions resided within the confines of the traditional medical literature. Thus, I dusted off my *Harrison's Text Book of Internal Medicine,* leafed through the index, and found references to vitamins. What I discovered was really not surprising at all. Although a two-page chart describing the many disastrous consequences of profound vitamin insufficiency was there, not much more was available to help me understand the consequences of minimal vitamin inadequacy and the many benefits of vitamin supplementation. I was perplexed. My prior "bible" of internal medicine had failed me. Where was I to turn?

The answer lay in a realm so foreign to me and most of my colleagues that the mere consideration of journeying into it sent shivers up and down my spine. This new world was that of natural medicine—a place few traditional doctors will even discuss, let alone visit.

I made my landing where you might expect, in the alternative medicine sections of bookstores and at various local health food stores. After devouring stacks of books on natural medicine, I began to communicate more intelligently with local health food store owners. "Hanging out" at these stores, I absorbed a great deal of information, both scientific and anecdotal. Barraging unsuspecting store owners with countless questions, I obtained numerous leads on my continuing quest for knowledge in this new world. My most valued guide on my evolving journey was *The Encyclopedia of Nutritional Supplements* by Michael T. Murray, N.D. I owe much to both Dr. Michael Murray and his mentor, Dr. Joe Pizzorno, the president and founder of Bastyr University, a naturopathic college. Without them and their numerous well-written and comprehensive texts, my journey would have been immeasurably more difficult.

With my new foundation of knowledge in how to use nutrients to combat disease, I expanded my studies to formulate my own cardiovascular vitamin, mineral, and nutrient supplement program. Here I will describe some of the more valuable supplements available for cardiovascular patients, or patients with cardiovascular risk factors. The absence of other vitamins and nutrients from our current discussion does not imply their unimportance.

I recommend vitamins and supplements to patients based on their symptoms and medical history; I do not, at present, perform tests to determine exact vitamin levels. The tests that currently exist are both quite expensive and incomplete. This is an evolving field, and hopefully these tests will become more refined, affordable, and common in the near future.

To understand why vitamins are important, a word about free radicals and antioxidants is a must. Free radicals are hyperreactive and potentially damaging substances which can be produced through *normal* metabolic processes in our bodies. Free radicals can be likened to the wildly speeding bouncing ball in the old video game "Breakout": As the ball randomly zips along the screen, it destroys anything it touches. Similarly, when free radicals are formed, they bounce furiously and at alarming speeds into neighboring molecules, altering and at times destroying them. Thus it is imperative that our bodies possess healthy defenses against their attack (and even their creation).

Enter the antioxidants. These wonderful substances represent our bodies' army, constantly limiting the formation of free radicals and fighting them back when they develop. Glutathione peroxidase, superoxide dismutase, vitamins E and C, coenzyme Q-10, and alpha lipoic acid are just a few of these marvelous warriors. Knowing the power of antioxidants, one would suspect at first glance that consuming huge quantities of them might render us immune to the free radical onslaught. Unfortunately, this is not necessarily the case. It turns out that antioxidants can themselves *transiently* become *weak* free radicals when they "do their jobs." These altered antioxidants are then reconverted to their superior state.

This cascade of antioxidants represents an intricate network that we do not yet completely understand. Consequently, we are still unsure of the "perfect" dosage recommendations for them. Too much can theoretically result in the formation of weak free radicals (i.e., altered antioxidants). Too little, and we leave ourselves open to the bombardment of powerful and damaging free radicals, which can lead to illnesses and possible early aging. Through my review of the literature and based on my clinical experience, I present here a dosage range for numerous minerals and vitamins, including the antioxidants. My belief is that a proper *balance* of antioxidants will prevent their permanent conversion into free radicals. Although I believe I have offered an appropriate and health-promoting dosage schedule, more investigation needs to be done to confirm my (and everybody else's) recommendations. I am in the process of establishing some of these studies. Hopefully, as the field of integrative medicine burgeons, we will know for certain *exactly* how much of each supplement we should take to maintain and restore health. For now, we must do the best we can with the data we have.

Vitamins

Vitamins are substances that enable enzymatic systems in our bodies to function appropriately. Because we lack the capacity to create vitamins, we have to consume them in our daily diet. Most people—even doctors—will admit that severe vitamin deficiencies can result in illness. Scurvy, a vitamin C deficiency, is the classic example. In the absence of vitamin C, collagen, a supporting structure of many of our tissues, cannot be formed. The result: bleeding gums, easy bruisability, and ineffective wound repair.

While we all agree that the absence of various vitamins can result in severe ailments, there is much debate with regard to the issue of an appropriate minimum dietary intake of vitamins and minerals. What vitamin and mineral intakes are needed to avoid mineral and vitamin deficiency? To address this matter, the Food and Nutrition

Board of the National Research Council has been establishing guidelines for Recommended Dietary Allowances (RDAs) since 1941. Surprisingly, the RDAs represent the minimum quantities of various vitamins and minerals required to keep 95 percent of all *healthy* Americans from developing overt vitamin deficiencies. The RDA does not address any individuals with medical illnesses such as hypertension, diabetes, or high cholesterol. It does not address the elderly, those consuming large quantities of alcohol, or those who continue to smoke cigarettes. Thus, the RDA has an extremely limited utility. It does not address situations in which, because of various disease conditions, an individual requires a markedly increased amount of a vitamin. As a result, the RDA should be used only as a dietary guide for the young and completely healthy.

Nevertheless, 5 percent of the people even in that population are still potential candidates for disorders caused by vitamin insufficiency. To further illustrate the inadequacy of the RDA, I will share a personal story.

The other day, my 9-year-old son, Jason, was exploring the computer. He has a wonderful CD which contains the entire encyclopedia Encarta. One of its many programs allows him to calculate his daily intake of various vitamins and minerals. To my son's surprise, his intake of thiamin fell below the RDA. To appreciate the substance of this discovery, you need to know that my son is not a typical 9-year-old—he eats a more well-rounded diet than most American adults. When we go out to dinner, he doesn't look for hot dogs and hamburgers; instead he inquires about the fish of the day. Thus, the realization that he was consuming too little thiamin was surprising, not just for him, but for me as well—of course, I had assumed his diet was more than adequate, or I would already have addressed its possible deficiencies. Fortunately, the simple addition of a vitamin supplement rectified his dietary shortcome.

Jason's discovery reinforced my belief that all Americans require vitamin supplementation. I also feel strongly that the RDA should not be used as a guide to determine appropriate quantities of vitamins and minerals. It is not only inadequate, but misleading, lulling many Americans into a false sense of confidence about their nutritional well-being.

Vitamin A and the Carotenoids

Of the four fat-soluble vitamins, A, D, E, and K, vitamin A was discovered first. By 1913, we understood vitamin A was an essential growth factor, and seventeen years later in 1930 researchers described its chemical structure. Because some of the carotenes can actually be converted into vitamin A, they are often grouped together with this vitamin. Carotenes, also called "carotenoids," are plant pigments possessing many wonderful health-promoting benefits. Over 600 carotenoids have already been described and the number continues to grow. Being fat-soluble, vitamin A and the carotenoids can be stored by the body, mostly in the liver. The body's ability to store any vitamin always raises the possibility of vitamin excess, so we must be cautious about recommending large quantities of the fat-soluble vitamins.

Vitamin A and the carotenes are believed to help limit the development of coronary disease—perhaps because they function as antioxidants.

We also know that vitamin A and beta carotene are extremely susceptible to oxidative damage; thus, when consumed in high doses along with oxidative stressors such as tobacco and alcohol, they can be potentially damaging. Nonetheless, individuals should not cease taking vitamin A and beta carotene supplements with doses ranging from 5,000 to 10,000 IU per day, in conjunction with smoking cessation, a limitation of alcohol intake, and concomitant use of other antioxidants. It is important to realize that there are also numerous noncardiac benefits of vitamin A and the carotenoids to the skin, eyes, and immune system.

Vitamin E

Vitamin E became popularized as the "antisterility" vitamin after a 1922 research team demonstrated that the absence of vitamin E resulted in infertility. This reputation led to the name "alpha tocopherol" being bestowed on the most active form of vitamin E, which means "to bear children" in Greek. Recently, as the many cardiovascular benefits of vitamin E have come to light, the brand of being the fertility vitamin has been lost. Since it is incorporated into our cell membranes, vitamin E acts as a sentinel guarding the integrity of our cells and ensuring their health and stability. In fact, vitamin E helps to prevent oxidative damage to LDL and other fat particles that otherwise would ultimately lead to the development of coronary artery disease. Numerous studies have established the cardiovascular benefits of vitamin E, and now even "traditional" cardiologists advocate its use. Vitamin E consumption has clearly been shown to decrease the risk of cardiovascular disease in both men and women. In addition to its salubrious role as an antioxidant, vitamin E possesses the added attributes of raising HDL levels and decreasing platelet stickiness. The Cambridge Heart Antioxidant Study (CHAOS), one of the best to demonstrate vitamin E's cardiovascular benefits, evaluated over 2,000 patients with coronary artery disease. Completed in 1996, this study demonstrated a greater than 75 percent reduction in the risk of heart attacks in patients treated with vitamin E.

Even in light of the substantial scientific evidence supporting its use, there are those who still underscore the possible side effects of vitamin E. Some people claim that vitamin E substantially increases the risk of bleeding. Having completed a thorough search of the literature, I have failed to find any studies that clearly demonstrate this finding. In fact, some studies seem to indicate that vitamin E may make bleeding less likely. In my own clinical experience, I have seen hundreds, if not thousands, of patients consume large quantities of vitamin E. Not once have I witnessed an adverse bleeding reaction caused by this invaluable nutrient. Thus, I believe that whether or not you are taking aspirin or Coumadin, vitamin E should be a part of your daily regimen as a means of limiting cardiovascular disease. My customary recommendation is 600 IU daily.

Vitamin E is also potentially beneficial in treating ailments such as fibrocystic breast disease, menopausal hot flashes, osteoarthritis, and Raynaud's phenomenon. Please remember when taking a vitamin E supplement: Not all vitamin Es are created equal. Ensure that yours is 100 percent Natural, D alpha tocopherol, *not* D, L alpha tocopherol (synthetic). The Natural form is clearly superior to the synthetic.

Vitamin C

Vitamin C is the most important of the water-soluble vitamins, acting as the first line of our bodies' defense against free radical attack.

Citrus fruits are the most celebrated sources of vitamin C. I gleefully recall Edith Bunker in *All in the Family* announcing that she always drinks her entire glass of orange juice because she never knows which half the vitamin C is in. Less commonly recognized is the fact that vitamin C is also present in substantial quantities in many vegetables, including broccoli, brussels sprouts, peppers, and potatoes.

Several of vitamin C's biological effects can limit cardiovascular disease. Vitamin C has been shown to lower cholesterol and triglycerides and raise high density lipoprotein cholesterol (HDL). Possibly by promoting the excretion of lead, vitamin C also lowers blood pressure levels. In addition, vitamin C also possesses the favorable effect of decreasing platelet stickiness. The most well-recognized cardiovascular utility of vitamin C, however, lies in its ability to function as a potent water-soluble antioxidant. Studies examining the cardiovascular benefits of vitamin C have been impressive. An epidemiologic evaluation performed at UCLA demonstrated that men who consumed over 300 mg of vitamin C daily lived about six years longer than those who took no vitamin C supplements. A Tufts University study demonstrated that people who consumed more than 700 mg of vitamin C daily had a 62 percent reduction in their risk of cardiovascular mortality. For optimum protection, I generally recommend that my heart patients take between 1,000 and 2,000 mg of vitamin C in divided doses daily.

As with most other vitamins, vitamin C has a huge spectrum of health benefits—enhancing immune function, improving tissue healing, and perhaps even limiting a variety of cancers. Even the FDA recognizes that smokers require at least twice the RDA in order to help limit the detrimental effects of tobacco abuse. This, of course, does not mean that one should continue smoking while simply adding vitamin C to his or her regimen. Smoking kills, and those who continue this deadly habit are either blind or shortsighted.

Niacin

Niacin—vitamin B_3—is *strictly speaking* not a vitamin, since it can be created within our bodies from tryptophan. As with all other vitamins, niacin functions in a multitude of enzymatic reactions, helping to keep us healthy and fit. Excellent food sources of niacin include organ meats, fish, and eggs. Niacin is a favorite of cardiologists because of its various cardiovascular benefits. It has been shown to lower levels of LDL, lipoprotein a, triglycerides, and fibrinogen. It has also been demonstrated to be one of the most effective agents at increasing HDL levels.

Although niacin clearly possesses cardiovascular benefits, it is not a drug for everyone. Patients with diabetes, gout, preexisting liver disease, a history of peptic ulcer disease, and even glaucoma should be cautious about ingesting large doses of niacin. When taking niacin in "therapeutic" doses of 1,500 to 3,000 mg daily, liver function tests to ensure your safety are a must. One of the most troubling side effects of niacin is a sense of flushing, which can make you feel as if you're on fire. This side effect is produced by the release of prostaglandins from blood vessels, so premedication with aspirin or Motrin-like medications (prostaglandin inhibitors) can often prevent its manifestation.

Inositol hexaniacinate, or No Flush Niacin, is an over-the-counter form of B_3 which does not result in flushing, and only very rarely causes liver problems. Unfortunately, No Flush Niacin is much less effective at lowering cholesterol and raising HDL. So, when treating very abnormal cholesterol levels, I choose another form of niacin, Niaspan, a long-acting preparation made by KOS Pharmaceuticals. Niaspan is effective and relatively well tolerated; I have had good results using it with my patients.

I must emphasize my conviction that the daily consumption of any form of extremely high-dose niacin is tantamount to taking a medication, and requires a physician's supervision. When used properly, however, niacin is a wonderful addition to many patients' vitamin routines.

Folic Acid

Folic acid, another B vitamin, is the most commonly deficient vitamin in the world. The reason for its rampant deficiency rests in the fact that foods high in folic acid—plant products—are not quite so frequently consumed as those low in folic acid, animal products. Alcohol also contributes to folic acid deficiency by impairing its metabolism. From a cardiac standpoint, folic acid's importance lies in the fact that it decreases levels of homocysteine, a protein by-product known to cause coronary artery disease. Folic acid is inexpensive and harmless, and in view of its tremendous cardiovascular benefit, I generally recommend that people take 1,000 mcg a day.

Vitamin B$_6$

Pyridoxine, or vitamin B$_6$, possesses a wide spectrum of therapeutic benefits. B$_6$'s benefit in treating (and preventing) cardiovascular disease was first documented by Killmer McCulley, M.D., in the late 1960s. Dr. McCulley demonstrated that B$_6$ supplementation will often help lower homocysteine levels. Other potential cardiovascular benefits include vitamin B$_6$'s ability to diminish platelet aggregation, lower blood pressure, and even lower cholesterol levels. Although B$_6$ is an extremely safe supplement, there have a been a few reports in the literature of possible toxicity from doses as low as 150 mg a day. Thus, I do not recommend prolonged consumption of over 150 mg of vitamin B$_6$ daily. For the purpose of homocysteine reduction, and for general adult supplementation, I recommend 50 mg as an appropriate daily dosage of pyridoxine.

Vitamin B$_6$ has also been shown to be helpful in the treatment of carpal tunnel syndrome, asthma, depression, diabetes, kidney stones, and in the prevention of "Chinese restaurant syndrome" (a result of consuming MSG).

Vitamin B$_{12}$

Vitamin B$_{12}$, or cobalamin, is the third and final B vitamin beneficial for reducing homocysteine levels (which have recently been recognized as posing a risk for the development of coronary artery disease). This substance has a unique place in the vitamin kingdom in that it is present in worthwhile amounts only in *animal* products. Fruits and vegetables contain minimal quantities of vitamin B$_{12}$. Although substances like tempeh may possess a small quantity of B$_{12}$, it is generally considered insufficient for our bodies' needs. Therefore, my personal advice is that all patients, especially those who are strict vegetarians, take a daily supplement of between 400 and 1,000 mcg of vitamin B_{12}. While it's not necessary to take vitamin B_{12} sublingually (under the tongue) to obtain its benefits, the vitamin is widely available in this form. In my opinion, most individuals will absorb sufficient amounts of vitamin B_{12} in its oral form, and therefore do not require additional B_{12} in a sublingual, or even injectable, preparation.

Pantethine

Pantethine, an active and stable—but expensive—form of vitamin B_5, has been shown to aid in the control of lipid abnormalities. Studies have shown that a dose of 300 mg three times a day can significantly diminish levels of triglycerides, LDL, and total cholesterol while producing the added benefit of elevating HDL levels. As its mode of action involves fatty acid transport and metabolism, pantethine works extremely well when used in combination with L-carnitine and coenzyme Q-10. I have often used pantethine in conjunction with these substances when treating hypercholesterolemic patients who either cannot or will not use conventional drug therapy.

Choline

Choline, a member of the B vitamin class, is an essential component of all our cell membranes. Choline, like pantethine, is critical in the metabolism of fats. It is found in legumes and egg yolks, primarily in the form of "phosphatidyl choline." Choline is beneficial in reducing cholesterol. Numerous German studies have demonstrated significant drops in triglyceride and total cholesterol levels and concomitant significant elevations in HDL levels with the administration of 1–3 grams of phosphatidyl choline daily. Because of the occasional problem of nausea and abdominal bloating, I have not utilized phosphatidyl choline on a large enough scale to assess its efficacy accurately. I am sure, though, that as more and more patients seek alternative modes of treating their cholesterol abnormalities, I will be able to gain a better grasp on this important vitamin's applicability.

Choline is also useful in managing liver disease and various neurologic abnormalities, such as Alzheimer's disease.

TABLE 23

How Cholesterol May Be Affected by Cholesterol-Lowering Supplements

↓ indicates that the supplement lowers the cholesterol component in question,
↑ indicates that the supplement increases its levels, and ⇔ indicates that the
supplement has no effect.

Supplement	Action
Vitamin C	↓ Total cholesterol ⇔ LPa ↑ HDL ⇔ LDL ⇔ Triglycerides
Niacin	↓ Total cholesterol ↓ LPa ↑ ↑HDL ↓ LDL ↓ Triglycerides
Pyridoxine	↓ Total cholesterol ⇔ LPa ↑ HDL ⇔ LDL ⇔ Triglycerides
Pantethine	↓ Total cholesterol ⇔ LPa ↑ HDL ↓ LDL ↓↓ Triglycerides
Choline	↓ Total cholesterol ⇔ LPa ↑ HDL ⇔ LDL ↓ Triglycerides
Chromium	↓ Total cholesterol ⇔ LPa ↑ HDL ⇔ LDL ↓ Triglycerides
L-carnitine	↓ Total cholesterol ⇔ LPa ↑ HDL ⇔ LDL ↓ Triglycerides

TABLE 23 (Continued)
How Cholesterol May Be Affected by Cholesterol-Lowering Supplements

Supplement	Action
Soluble fiber	↓ Total cholesterol ⇔ LPa ⇔ HDL ↓ LDL ⇔ Triglycerides
Cayenne pepper	↓ Total cholesterol ⇔ LPa ⇔ HDL ⇔ LDL ↓ Triglycerides
Garlic	↓ Total cholesterol ⇔ LPa ↑ HDL ↓ LDL ↓ Triglycerides
Gugulipid	↓ Total cholesterol ⇔ LPa ↑ HDL ↓ LDL ↓ Triglycerides
Panax ginseng	↓ Total cholesterol ⇔ LPa ↑ HDL ↓ LDL ↓ Triglycerides
Turmeric	↓ Total cholesterol ⇔ LPa ↑ HDL ↓ LDL ↓ Triglycerides
Soy	↓ Total cholesterol ⇔ LPa ⇔ HDL ⇔ LDL ↓ Triglycerides

TABLE 23 (Continued)
How Cholesterol May Be Affected by Cholesterol-Lowering Supplements

Omega-3 fatty acids (DHA and EPA)	↓ Total cholesterol
	⇔ LPa
	⇔ HDL
	⇔ LDL
	↓↓ Triglycerides

Minerals

Minerals, like vitamins, are required in small quantities in order to satisfy the needs of our enzymatic machinery. When more than 100 mg of a given mineral are required on a daily basis, it is defined as a major mineral; the need for less than 100 mg a day defines a minor mineral. In total, there are eighteen minerals needed for proper human functioning—seven are major, and eleven are minor. Several minerals possess considerable relevance in treating and preventing cardiovascular disease.

Magnesium

Of all the minerals employed in the treatment of cardiovascular disease, magnesium is far and away my favorite. Unfortunately, most Americans are probably deficient in this vital substance. While the RDA for magnesium is 350 mg, it has been found that the average American consumes merely 143–266 mg a day. Magnesium is found in great quantities in food substances such as tofu, seeds, nuts, and whole grains. Yet Americans are generally averse to consuming this kind of diet. So why should we worry about magnesium deficiency, what does magnesium do, and what happens to us when we lack it?

Magnesium, like many other minerals and vitamins, is involved in the activation of numerous enzyme systems within our bodies, including those impacting the cardiovascular system. If you refer to Chapter 6, you will find a review of magnesium's utility in treating acute heart attacks. The bottom line is that when magnesium is administered early, it probably can significantly limit the devastation of a heart attack.

Described as the body's "natural calcium channel blocker," magnesium has been utilized in the treatment of angina and high blood pressure (hypertension). I have witnessed its beneficial effects in treating patients with both of these conditions. The most dramatic and rewarding benefit of magnesium that I have noted, however, is in treating patients with palpitations and minor heart rhythm disturbances.

One of the most frustrating disorders to treat, from a cardiologist's perspective, is palpitations. Most medications aimed at the elimination of this symptom are toxic. Of the natural approaches, including taurine, the essential fatty acids, coenzyme Q-10, and magnesium, my experience has revealed magnesium to be king. It is truly wonderful to witness the dramatic responses of many patients to this simple mineral. I would estimate that three-quarters of the patients I've treated with magnesium have found their palpitations to be either completely eliminated or markedly improved.

One study, in fact, has demonstrated that magnesium offered patients a significant benefit in the treatment of new-onset atrial fibrillation. Magnesium is also the treatment of choice for a life-threatening rhythm disturbance called *torsade de pointes*—often the *consequence* of *anti-arrhythmic medications*—which can lead to fainting or even death. Patients who are fortunate enough to make it alive to the hospital are immediately admitted to the intensive care unit and treated with—of all things—intravenous magnesium. Usually the abnormal rhythm will miraculously melt away as magnesium is infused into the patient's vein. A magnesium infusion—a simple and "natural" therapy—represents a great advance over the previous employment of temporary pacemakers in the treatment of *torsade de pointes*. Thus, unwittingly, physicians have begun to incorporate gifts of nature into their everyday practice of medicine.

Magnesium plays a major role in the treatment of a noncardiac but vascular disorder: intermittent claudication, a painful cramping of the legs caused by blockages in the blood vessels feeding the lower extremities. This condition afflicts nearly 10 percent of the elderly population. Numerous natural remedies are available for the treatment of this painful condition, including L-carnitine, coenzyme Q-10, vitamin E, ginkgo biloba, and the essential fatty acids. Magnesium also contributes greatly to the relief of pain which plagues these patients. Studies of claudication patients have documented their very low magnesium levels, and the administration of magnesium supplements to these patients results in a significant improvement in their symptoms. In light of magnesium's common deficiency among Americans, and its clear benefit in the treatment of many disorders—cardiovascular and otherwise—I strongly recommend daily supplementation with at least 250 mg. As long as you are not suffering from kidney disease, more is probably better. Be careful, however, when starting magnesium, as it can have the side effect of diarrhea. I would, therefore, recommend starting your regimen with 300 mg a day. If you do not develop diarrhea (which would be unusual at this low dose), continue or increase the dose, if necessary. Please also be aware that the chelated forms of magnesium, such as glycinate or citrate, are both less likely to cause diarrhea and are better absorbed than the inorganic form such as oxide.

In addition, magnesium is beneficial in a variety of noncardiovascular disease processes. For instance, magnesium, especially when used in conjunction with vitamin B_6, can diminish the production of kidney stones in those patients susceptible to stone formation. When used for stone reduction, magnesium citrate is probably its most advantageous form. Magnesium has also been helpful in the treatment of migraine headaches. Andrea Peralta, the transcriptionist who has done such a wonderful job working with me on this book, has suffered from migraines for many years. The addition of magnesium to her daily vitamin intake resulted in a significant decrease in the frequency of her migraine headaches. Another noncardiac disorder considered to be related to magnesium depletion is PMS. A plague for many women, PMS is at least partially caused by low magnesium levels. The supplementation of magnesium may help limit this extremely troubling disorder.

Calcium

Calcium, the most plentiful mineral in the body, resides almost exclusively in our bones. This mineral, as with others, is an integral component of many enzymatic processes. It serves a critical function in maintaining normal heart and skeletal muscle activity, plays a role in the proper clotting of our blood, and is an essential component of neurotransmitter release. Although milk is often considered the best source of calcium, plant substances like tofu, spinach, and kale also contain large quantities of calcium. I was shocked to discover that kale is actually a better source of calcium than milk, since its calcium is more "bioavailable."

Calcium's impact on blood pressure is an area of great interest for both the cardiologist and the heart disease patient. Overall, the results of various studies have been inconsistent. It is now felt that certain patients who are "salt sensitive," such as African-Americans and the elderly, may experience a blood pressure–lowering benefit with the supplementation of calcium. If you decide to take calcium supplements, be careful to purchase one that does not contain lead. Dolomite and bone meal products are two types of calcium supplements that have been historically loaded with lead, so you should avoid them. Having the lowest concentrations of lead and being best absorbed, calcium carbonate or calcium that has been chelated to substances such as citrate or gluconate (the bottle's label will say, "calcium gluconate" or "calcium citrate") are probably your best options.

Zinc

The most ubiquitous of all minerals, zinc is involved in more enzymatic reactions than any other mineral substance. It is also a component of every cell in our bodies, and thus has an expansive impact on our bodies. Its deficiency can result in diarrhea, changes in our skin, loss of hair, recurrent infections, mental disturbances, and prostate problems. People prone to the development of zinc deficiency include vegetarians, diabetics, alcoholics, and patients on hemodialysis. Although there is no single cardiovascular disorder that requires zinc supplementation, it is essential for proper heart function. Therefore, I recommend a daily zinc intake of between 20 and 30 mg.

Copper

Following iron and zinc, copper is the third most abundant of the trace minerals. Lysyl-oxidase, an enzyme essential in the cross-linking of collagen and elastin (providing structural integrity for our arteries and other tissues), is dependent upon copper for its proper functioning. An abnormality in this enzyme system will result in bone and joint disorders, as well as weakened blood vessel walls. Lipid abnormalities also develop with copper deficiency. LDL will be elevated and HDL, the protective cholesterol, will be reduced. Thus it is imperative for cardiovascular patients to maintain proper copper levels. Since zinc decreases copper's absorption, copper dosage is dependent upon that of zinc. It is generally recommended that one consume zinc and copper in a ratio of 10:1. For patients suffering from vascular abnormalities, especially aortic and other aneurysms, I strongly advise the consumption of adequate amounts of copper, in the range of 2 to 3 mg daily.

Potassium

Potassium is a major mineral that is critical to the health of all cells. It is crucial to the proper functioning of our nervous systems, and to the electrical excitability of our hearts. To keep our heart's electrical "wiring" healthy (and the rest of our bodies, too), we should consume a diet in which the ratio of potassium to sodium is 5:1. Unfortunately, the typical American diet is much higher in sodium than in potassium—1 part potassium to 2 parts sodium—which can lead to high blood pressure and other problems. Because potassium imbalance (deficiency or excess) can result in serious, even life-threatening, consequences (such as causing the heart not to beat at the proper rhythm or speed), supplements are limited to 99 mg by law. Good food sources of potassium include green leafy vegetables, fruits (especially bananas), and legumes.

Selenium

A minor mineral, selenium is a crucial component of the antioxidant enzyme glutathione peroxidase, and it works with vitamin E to protect cell membranes. Decreased selenium levels have been correlated with the development of not only cardiovascular disease, but also cancer. Selenium supplementation increases HDL cholesterol and decreases platelet aggregation. To protect themselves from both cardiovascular disease and cancer, it's particularly important for smokers to supplement with selenium. Brazil nuts are the food that is highest in selenium. I recommend supplementing with no more than 800 mcg daily. At times, it is easy to determine whether the dose you're taking is too high for you, because selenium toxicity produces a distinctive "garlic breath," nausea, and nail and hair breakage.

Selenium deficiency has been most clearly linked to the development of both cardiovascular disease and arthritis in studies performed in a part of China in which the soil is particularly selenium-depleted (and the people are too poor to supplement, even if supplements are available). Young women and children were found to be the most severely affected.

Other Helpful Supplements

L-Carnitine

L-carnitine, the rogue child of the amino acids and vitamins, fits into no easy category. There are those who claim it is a vitamin, yet it is produced in our bodies and thus, strictly speaking, cannot be considered a vitamin. Since it lacks an amine group, it cannot be called an amino acid. It is, however, synthesized from the amino acid lysine, causing many people erroneously to refer to L-carnitine as an amino acid itself.

However it is classified, L-carnitine is a wonderful supplement endowed with many cardiovascular benefits. It functions like no other natural or pharmaceutical agent. By facilitating the transport of fatty acids across mitochondrial membranes, L-carnitine enables muscles—both skeletal and heart—to function at improved levels even in the absence of an adequate oxygen supply. Thus, people suffering from claudication or angina can achieve great relief by consuming L-carnitine.

It gives me great pleasure to help people with claudication by using natural supplements. Claudication is a painful sensation in the lower extremities which occurs with walking. It is caused by a reduction of blood flow because of arterial blockages. Over 80 percent of the patients with this disorder that I've treated have enjoyed dramatic improvements when given carnitine at a dose of 2 g twice a day. Other supplements which add to L-carnitine's success are vitamin E, coenzyme Q-10, magnesium, the essential fatty acids, and ginkgo biloba. L-carnitine is also beneficial in treating acute heart attack (myocardial infarction), and studies have demonstrated that it improves patients' recovery. In addition, L-carnitine can improve heart muscle function in patients suffering from congestive heart failure. Another salutary effect of L-carnitine is its impact on serum lipids. Working very well in combination with pantethine, L-carnitine has been shown to lower triglycerides and total cholesterol levels while raising the heart-saving HDL. In *The Carnitine Miracle,* author Robert Crayhon repeatedly reinforces the fact that most Americans are deficient in L-carnitine. Unfortunately, the best source of L-carnitine is red meat. While Americans are attempting to improve their health by limiting red meat consumption, they are unwittingly limiting the intake of this essential nutrient. I advise (as does Mr. Crayhon) that patients consume at least 250 mg of supplemental carnitine daily.

Coenzyme Q-10

Coenzyme Q-10 (co-Q-10) exists in every cell in the body, and thus is called ubiquinone. It is an essential component of our energy-producing mitochondria, and so is integrally connected with L-carnitine. As opposed to L-carnitine, which is found mostly in meats, coenzyme Q-10's primary source is plants. Coenzyme Q-10 possesses a variety of cardiovascular benefits. It is one of very few substances valuable in managing mitral valve prolapse—a generally benign, but often troubling disorder resistant to the effects of most pharmaceutical agents. Several studies have also documented the blood pressure–lowering benefit of coenzyme Q-10. This effect is not well understood and requires at least four months of continuous supplementation to occur. A fascinating study assessing coronary artery bypass surgery patients demonstrated beneficial effects of coenzyme Q-10 through the pretreatment of these surgical patients. By giving patients 150 mg of co-Q-10 daily for seven days prior to surgery, oxidative damage was reduced. I advocate its use in all patients who are about to undergo coronary artery bypass grafting.

One of the most impressive uses of coenzyme Q-10 is in the treatment of congestive heart failure. As you may recall, congestive heart failure can be a devastating condition resulting in not only a limitation of activity level, but also a reduction of life span. Steven Sinatra, M.D., a cardiologist practicing in Connecticut, is one of the greatest

TABLE 24
Supplements That Help Manage Cardiac Conditions

Condition	Helpful Supplement (Daily Dosage)
Coronary artery disease	Magnesium (300 mg) Vitamin E (400–800 IU) Coenzyme Q-10 (100 mg) Omega-3 fatty acids (2,000-3,000 mg) L-carnitine (250–500 mg twice daily)
Congestive heart failure	Vitamin E (400-800 IU) Coenzyme Q-10 (100–400 mg) Magnesium (300 mg) Omega-3 fatty acids (2,000-3,000 mg) L-carnitine (1–2 g twice daily) Hawthorn extract (approximately 400 mg)
Excessive clotting	Omega-3 fatty acids (2,000-3,000 mg) Vitamin E (400-800 IU) Ginkgo biloba (180 mg) Grape seed extract (40 mg) Garlic (4,000 mcg) Selenium (800 mcg or less)
Claudication (leg pain due to blocked arteries)	L-carnitine (2 g twice daily) Vitamin E (400–800 IU) Coenzyme Q-10 (100 mg) Magnesium (300–600 mg) Omega-3 fatty acids (2,000-3,000 mg) Ginkgo biloba (180 mg)
High blood pressure	Vitamin C (1,000–2,000 mg) Calcium (300 mg twice daily) Hawthorn extract (approximately 400 mg) Coleus (150 mg) Khella (200 mg) Garlic (4,000 mcg)
Arrhythmias	Magnesium (300–600 mg) Potassium (99 mg) and potassium-rich foods L-taurine (3 grams) EPA/DHA (3,000 mg) Coenzyme Q-10 (100-200 mg) Hawthorn extract (approximately 400 mg)
Palpitations	Magnesium (300–600 mg) Omega-3 fatty acids (2,000–3,000 mg) Coenzyme Q-10 (100 mg)

proponents of coenzyme Q-10. He has performed a multitude of studies utilizing coenzyme Q-10 to treat heart failure patients. Because of his advice (and the results of numerous scientific studies), I have used this supplement in my own heart failure patients at doses as high as 400 mg daily. Although I do not have a large enough series of patients to document statistically significant improvements in heart muscle function, I can tell you that my heart failure patients do *feel* much better when taking coenzyme Q-10.

I have also witnessed "objective" improvement in heart muscle function in severely compromised patients consuming large doses of co-Q-10. Recently, for example, after taking of 400 mg daily of co-Q-10 for one year, a patient of mine suffering from coronary artery disease had an ECHO cardiogram documenting a dramatic improvement in his heart muscle function. In fact, his ejection fraction (normal being greater than or equal to 55 percent) soared from 20 percent to 50 percent. This rarely observed change resulted not only in an amelioration of his symptoms, but in a clearly definable change in his heart muscle, which can translate into longer life.

Since co-Q-10 is such a vital substance, it is important for physicians to realize that several drugs used in the treatment of heart patients can actually lower its levels. Beta blockers, statins, and oral hypoglycemic agents have all been shown to decrease coenzyme Q-10 levels. In patients taking these drugs, at least 30 mg co-Q-10 a day is required to replenish this lost supply. Broad-based dosage recommendations are difficult. I vary the dosage of co-Q-10 depending on the ailment being treated. I do recommend, however, that a daily baseline of 30 mg should be taken by all Americans.

And, yes, coenzyme Q-10 is also a potent antioxidant. It works hand-in-hand with vitamin E and other antioxidants to help prevent free radical damage to cell membranes and plasma lipids.

Alpha Lipoic Acid

As an antioxidant, there are few better than alpha lipoic acid, a sulfur-containing cofactor involved in the cellular production of energy. It is unique in being both water- and fat-soluble. Alpha lipoic acid is an important constituent of the antioxidant cascade which includes, among other antioxidants, vitamins E and C. This cascade represents a fascinating network of antioxidants which interact with one another in order to ensure their safety and longevity. Because of its critical role in this network and because of the knowledge that antioxidants are so crucial in the fight against heart disease, I recommend a small dose of alpha lipoic acid to all of my patients. A daily dose of 20 to 50 mg is a reasonable starting point. I would not advocate greater amounts until studies documenting the benefit of higher dosages are available. One special circumstance, however, in which higher doses may be indicated is in treating patients with diabetic neuropathies (pain or numbness from diabetes). Several studies have suggested that 2.00 mg three times a day may limit the pain of this disorder. I have tried this regimen in several patients and not found it to be effective. I do not mean to imply that this is a worthless treatment option, just that I have not yet observed its fruitfulness. More studies must be done in order to establish its place in the management of diabetic neuropathies.

Essential Fatty Acids

"Essential" fatty acids are fats which our bodies cannot produce. Because of our bodies' inability to manufacture these substances, we must consume them in order to remain healthy. It turns out that, as is the case with many other "good" things, we do not eat enough of the essential fatty acids. The spectrum of disorders which can result from essential fatty acid deficiency is enormous.

There are two principal essential fatty acids: an omega-3 fatty acid (alpha linolenic acid) and an omega-6 fatty acid (linoleic acid). A normal daily diet should maintain a ratio of 1:4 omega-3 to omega-6 fatty acids. The average American consumes a diet containing omega-3s and omega-6s in the ratio of between 1:20 to 1:40—a far cry from the health-promoting 1:4 ratio. We must all, therefore, increase our intake of the omega-3 fatty acids. Excellent food sources include flaxseed oil and cold water fish such as salmon, mackerel, herring, halibut, and trout. These fish contain the longer chain omega-3 fatty acids: EPA (eicosapentaenoic acid) and DHA (docosahexaenoic acid). The omega-3 fatty acid found in flax, alpha linolenic acid, can be partially converted by the body to EPA.

What wonderful cardiovascular benefits do these strangely named substances possess? First, the omega-3 fatty acids have been observed to lower total cholesterol and triglyceride levels. In my patients with high triglycerides, I have found the omega-3 fatty acids to be extraordinarily effective at lowering their levels. As many of my patients also have high blood pressure, supplementation with the omega-3 fatty acids has the added benefit of treating this disorder, significantly lowering their blood pressure (an effect that has also been documented in numerous studies). The omega-3 fatty acids have also been shown to diminish fibrinogen levels. Fibrinogen, you may recall from Chapter 4, is a component of blood that, when elevated, is associated with an increased risk of heart disease. As the omega-3 fatty acids lower fibrinogen levels, they will most likely decrease the risk of cardiovascular disease.

A side benefit of the omega-3 fatty acids is their utility in the treatment of arthritis. I recall one of my patients whom I had placed on an omega-3 fatty acid supplement because of elevated triglyceride levels and hypertension. Several weeks later the patient returned with a dramatically improved blood pressure reading. Even more importantly (from her perspective), she stated incredulously that her arthritis had resolved. She queried whether the omega-3 fatty acids were responsible. At the time, I was unaware of the importance of omega-3 fatty acids in the treatment of arthritis, so I did some research. Indeed, I discovered that the omega-3 and omega-6 fatty acids have been found to be extremely beneficial in the treatment of various inflammatory conditions such as arthritis.

Overall, I feel that the essential fatty acids are too often absent from the American diet, and should, therefore, be included in the daily regimen of all Americans. My nutritionist Nancy Szeman insists that all of our patients supplement their diets with essential fatty acids. After reviewing the literature, I feel that she is justified in her ardent support of this supplement.

Please be aware that any oil high in omega-3 or -6 fatty acids (polyunsaturated fats), such as flaxseed oil, is very easily damaged (oxidized). These fatty acids and the oils containing them should always be refrigerated, and never used in cooking, because heat destroys their health-giving properties. Also, when consuming these oils as supplements, you should always ensure that you are taking an adequate supply of the "oil-protective" vitamin E at a dose of 400–800 IU daily.

CHAPTER 12

Nature's Edible Gifts

Every autumn my wife, children, and I fly back to New York and New Jersey to revisit our roots. My wife, from New Jersey, and I, from New York, still have parents and siblings, nephews and nieces, and even one set of grandparents remaining in the tri-state region. Our children, although living over 1,000 miles away from their cousins, still possess a strong emotional connection to their relatives and eagerly await their annual sojourn. This past year, we began our trip in Woodcliff Lake, New Jersey, at my in-laws' home. A beautiful small town, Woodcliff Lake possesses many rustic characteristics. Homes are separated by acres, horse farms lie within walking distance, and trees and shrubbery abound. Our three days in Woodcliff Lake were wonderful. We took walks, enjoyed the open air, visited the horses, consumed fresh brown eggs, and felt fully relaxed.

The next leg of our trip was a journey to the jungle—New York City. Since my parents, brother, and sister still dwell in this cramped community of compartmentalized concrete, we tentatively traveled to the island of Manhattan. Although we know the many merits of Manhattan—shows, restaurants, and unparalleled diversity—our five senses were obviously troubled by our upcoming trip. Almost instantly, our five senses were inundated with input. The sounds, sight, and speed of the crowds of people and the cars barraged us. We struggled through the next three days, rushing to catch buses and subways, meeting family members uptown, downtown, crosstown; catching a movie here or there; and occasionally escaping into Central Park so we could see sunlight shimmering through the tall tree tops rather than being filtered by mountains of steel.

Although I had previously enjoyed eleven years of my life living in Manhattan, this trip was different. I apologize to the millions of Manhattan and other city dwellers for my apparent condemnation of city living, but I must be honest: We felt trapped, stifled, and at times, beaten by excessive input. I must clarify, though, that cities are simply external representations of what occurs in most of our "modern" lives, whether we dwell in Manhattan or Billings, Montana. The daily "hustle and bustle" of living—the balancing of families, friends, and competitive careers—reflects an internal chaos that affects all Americans trying to "get ahead." Having also just escaped from my own personal medley of professional stressors, I was poorly equipped to handle the overwhelming rush of midtown Manhattan.

After three days, we left the city and made our way to New Paltz, New York, where we stayed at the Mohunk Mountain House. This final leg of our trip was the home of my epiphany. A beautiful, secluded, and peaceful place, the mountain house appears to be etched into the side of a hill, and it overlooks a green mountain lake, surrounded by cleanly carved cliffs. We awoke each morning to sights so still and beautiful that even three screaming children could not steal our tranquility. Each day my wife, three small children, and I walked miles among cliffs, through back woods, along small streams and across smooth, grassy fields. An abundance of flowers, trees, and plants encased us. The air's clean, earthy smell mixed with the sun's soft filtered light permeated us.

I am not exaggerating when I tell you that my wife and I have never been more relaxed than we were during our stay at the Mohunk Mountain Lodge. Our emotional peace extended well beyond the sense of calm—our love and appreciation for our children and each other blossomed. We enjoyed and cherished each moment of our stay.

My epiphany may seem obvious, but what I learned from my stay in the mountains is that human beings are *intended* to be a part of nature. In fact, we are unmistakably one with nature. There is no question that the sounds, smells, sights, and embraces of the natural world are more healing and beneficial, more soothing and salubrious, than the sensual assaults of city dwelling. Although this is a simple truth, we often ignore it. We dismiss nature, separating ourselves from it as though we have evolved beyond it and no longer benefit from its gifts. We act as though nature were a parent that we have outgrown. By doing this, we deprive ourselves of nature's gifts—both spiritual and edible.

Through my experience at the Mohunk Mountain House, interlaced with the knowledge I have attained through readings about herbal medicine, my own personal understanding of man's place in the natural world has evolved. In the context of our million-year metamorphosis, our 100 years of modern urban living represents a mere split second. It is hubris that has harmfully caused us to believe we are distinct from nature. During human evolution, we grew side-by-side with plants, trees, flowers, birds, and animals. Natural selection enabled us to progress, maintaining and perpetuating our "better" attributes.

Natural selection, however, affects not only humankind but also all other living elements. I believe that humans, evolving side-by-side with plants and trees actually impacted on their evolution, and they on ours. When human beings ate vegetables or fruits possessing healthful characteristics, they would perhaps favor the plants producing them, help cultivate them, and in a sense lead to their continued survival.

This, of course, is an oversimplification, but I use it just to make a point. For millions of years, humans lived clearly within the context of nature, and for thousands of years nature was our only pharmaceutical repository. It has been only within the last 50 to 100 years—remember, this represents a mere blink of an eye in the context of our evolution—that we have been synthesizing drugs outside of nature in the scientific laboratory. Therefore, it should come as no surprise when I sing the songs of praise to medicinal herbs that human beings have benefitted from for the past 5,000 years.

In this chapter I will lay the groundwork of basic herbology principles and tell you about herbs possessing heart-health-promoting properties, so that you may come to enjoy their many benefits.

Herbs are traditionally defined as the aerial or aboveground portion of a plant that can be used for its medicinal, culinary, or perfuming attributes. There are five major categories of herbs—aromatic, astringent, bitter, mucilaginous, and nutritive.

Aromatic Herbs

The aromatic herbs possess high quantities of volatile oils. As these oils easily vaporize at room temperature, they release strong and characteristic odors. Aromatic herbs typically possess either stimulant or nervine (relaxing) effects. Ylang-ylang is a prototypical aromatic herb. When this herb's volatile oils penetrate the olfactory bulbs of the brain, waves of relaxation can be felt flowing through the body. Ylang-ylang also possesses a strong blood pressure–lowering effect, probably as a consequence of its intensely relaxing nature. Not knowing that my mother-in-law tends to have low blood pressure, I gave her a whiff of ylang-ylang, causing her nearly to faint on the spot. Fortunately, I had my trusty rosemary in hand—a stimulating aromatic herb—which, when sniffed, quickly counteracted ylang-ylang's blood pressure–lowering effects. My mother-in-law survived, and with the exception of some scars caused by a few choice words from my father-in-law, so too did I.

Orange, marjoram, patchouli, and clary sage essential oils also promote relaxation. Valerian, another aromatic herb (although it doesn't have as pleasant a smell—in fact, it's been described as smelling like dirty socks) contains chemicals called "valerotropes," which cause sedation. Thus, valerian is an herb commonly used for the treatment of insomnia.

Peppermint, an aromatic herb that's often brewed into tea, can both alleviate headaches and improve digestion.

Aromatic herbs can also be beneficial in the management of pain, fever, asthma, and sleep disorders. They are extremely safe and have relatively few contraindications.

Astringent Herbs

Astringent herbs owe their properties to tannins, a type of alcohol that interacts with proteins. These substances are best recognized for their role as leather tanners. They also endow great benefit to human beings (without tanning us). They have analgesic, antiseptic, and hemostatic properties, often being used in styptic pencils. They can usually be recognized by their bitter taste and frequently possess a constipating effect. Because of the way they interact with proteins, they can, unfortunately, impede the action of digestive enzymes. Therefore, astringent herbs should generally be avoided in patients with severe pancreatic disorders. Most other people, however, can tolerate these herbs without experiencing any significant side effects.

The active ingredient in aspirin, "salicylate," comes from white willow bark, an astringent herb that can be used as a painkiller (analgesic). White willow bark is actually a safer painkiller than aspirin, because it contains some mucilage that protects the stomach. Aspirin, as most people know, can cause severe gastrointestinal upset in susceptible individuals.

Bitter Herbs

Bitter herbs are the source of two powerful drugs that affect the heart: atropine speeds the heart rate and reserpine lowers blood pressure. These herbs owe their properties to a variety of substances: phenols, alkaloids, and saponins. Saponins are interesting substances in that they emulsify, or break down, oils. They derive their name from the Latin term *sapo*, which means soap. These agents can function as laxatives, expectorants, and even diuretics when consumed orally. The alkaloid-containing bitter herbs represent the most powerful of all plant constituents. Many modern and potentially toxic pharmacologic agents are derived from alkaloids. Although the alkaloid bitter herbs can be very useful, they also can be extremely dangerous and must be used with caution.

Two examples of commonly used bitter herbs are cascara and sarsaparilla. Cascara sagrada bark (a tree bark) is a bitter herb that can be used as a laxative. Sarsaparilla root's active ingredient is found in root beer foam. It can be used for skin diseases (like psoriasis), as an arthritis remedy, and also as a diuretic. Sarsaparilla root is not approved for these uses by the German Commission E (a very conservative organization), because of lack of proof that it actually works, not because of any risk.

Mucilaginous Herbs

Mucilage, a slimy substance comprised of sugar derivatives, can soothe and protect surfaces it comes into contact with. Mucilage can be used as emollients, agents which aid the skin, or demulcents, agents which mollify the GI tract and the throat. Mucilaginous herbs, which are generally not digested by the gastrointestinal tract and are therefore not absorbed into the body, exert no significant effects on our cardiovascular system. They can, however, soothe irritations of the stomach and duodenum. Slippery elm, a prototypical mucilaginous herb, is a wonderful agent for treating upset stomachs. Having successfully used this herb to settle my own stomach, I began suggesting it to many of my patients with the same ailment; they found it to be remarkably beneficial. Capsules of slippery elm can either be swallowed whole, or broken open and the contents ingested.

Aloe leaf is another mucilaginous herb that can be used as both a laxative and to soothe upset stomachs.

Nutritive Herbs

As you might expect, nutritive herbs are plants that have a medicinal effect while also providing proteins, carbohydrates, fats, vitamins, and minerals. The nutritive herb asparagus root, for instance, contains vitamins A, B_6, folic acid, and the minerals, copper, magnesium, and potassium. Spirulina algae contains chromium, iron, protein, manganese, zinc, and vitamins B_1, B_2, and B_3.

Rose hips fruit, an extraordinarily good source of vitamin C, was discovered by the Europeans during World War II. (Some of the vitamin C in rose hips fruit is unfortunately lost when it is processed into supplement form.) This nutritive herb also contains calcium and vitamins A, E, B_1, and B_2.

Although it is helpful to understand these five categories of herbs, one must not be lulled into a false sense of simplicity. Nature is not so easily compartmentalized. Herbs generally possess properties from more than one of these categories. They do, however, tend to have a dominant effect which lies within one of the five aforementioned groups. Since many of you will undoubtedly explore the benefits of herbs after completing this chapter, we should discuss the various forms in which herbs can be purchased.

When walking into a health food store for the first time, you may be drawn to the large jars of herbs lining a series of shelves. These jars can conjure images of old-time apothecaries and thus may seem to be saying, "Try me, taste me." Although making your own herbal preparation would be a wonderful experience, my advice to the novice herbalist is to avoid whole herbs.

If you are compelled to try them, however, there are several key elements to look for when selecting a dried herb sample. First there is the overall appearance of the sample. There must be clearly recognizable plant components and there should be minimal dust or dirt present. Second, the color must be as close to normal or natural as possible. Leaves should approximate their original green and flowers should maintain their natural colors. Any color loss implies sun-drying, prolonged storage, or poor storage conditions. Third, the smell is extremely important. An herb should smell fresh and clean, and if it is an aromatic sample, it should exude the strong aroma of its important constituents. Finally, there is the taste. In most circumstances, you should be able to taste a small piece of the herb and then quickly expectorate it. It should taste clean and distinctive. All expected tastes should be present and any unexpected taste should quickly alert the observer to possible adulterants. Having said this, I will reiterate that the novice herbalist should probably avoid obtaining dried herb samples until becoming more familiar with "appropriate" herb characteristics.

The two most commonly utilized forms of herbs include tinctures (liquid herb extractions) and dried standardized herbs in capsules. Tinctures are created by immersing herbs in liquid substances which then draw the important herbal constituents into the liquid. The tincture's strength is recognized by its concentration. A 1:5 tincture is 1 part herb, 5 parts liquid, and thus is weaker than a 1:1 tincture, which has equal parts herb and liquid. For those among us who cannot swallow pills, tinctures are preferred.

Alternatively, herbs can be dried and then standardized. This means that each capsule (or dropperful, if it's a liquid preparation) will contain the same amount of the herbal component that possesses a particular medical benefit. This standardization enables the consumer to have greater confidence in what he is purchasing. When buying an herb to treat a particular medical ailment, be sure you are getting a standardized extract from a reputable company.

Now let's discover some practical applications of a sampling of favorite herbs.

Herbs of Cardiovascular Appeal

Hawthorn (Crateagus)

Among the scores of herbs promoting cardiovascular health, I chose hawthorn as the one to lead me into the world of herbal medicine. Hawthorn was my preference as a ground-breaker chiefly because of its safety. In reviewing a substantial body of literature evaluating this herb, I found no references to any dangerous side effects. (In fact, limited research has suggested that adding hawthorn to patients receiving Digoxin can rarely result in a significant slowing of the heart rate. Ever-vigilantly I monitor my patients taking this combination, yet I have never seen this side effect.) I thus felt secure that I would not be harming my patients by administering hawthorn. Safety, though essential, in the absence of efficacy would be tantamount to administering a placebo here. Therefore, I also wanted my first herb to be one with documented beneficial effects.

Hawthorn is such an herb. The literature is replete with references to its benefits in the treatment of cardiovascular ailments. Studies have demonstrated hawthorn's blood pressure–lowering effect. It has been shown that coronary arteries can be meaningfully dilated with the administration of this herbal supplement. As hawthorn increases the heart's ability to contract (inotropy), it is also beneficial in treating mild congestive heart failure. Because of its combined safety and efficacy, I began to use hawthorn in the treatment not only of mild congestive heart failure, but also of more severe forms of this disease. Although the therapeutic value of hawthorn is difficult to state with absolute certainty in the absence of controlled clinical trials, my patients have responded favorably to this herb. I must confess, though, that through the years I have been recommending hawthorn in the form of berries or flowers.

While researching this book, I learned from the newly published *Complete German Commission E Monographs* by Blumenthal and colleagues that this may not be the wisest recommendation. The Commission E monographs present a German organization's exhaustive evaluations of a wide spectrum of herbs. Herbs are either "approved" or "unapproved" by Commission E, based upon the presence of side effects or a lack of substantial documentation of any clinical efficacy. I was shocked to discover that the only form of hawthorn which Commission E approved was an extract of hawthorn leaf with flower, consisting of dried flowering twig tips. Commission E found that this was the sole form of hawthorn that clearly possessed clinical benefit. Other formulations such as isolated berries, flowers, or leaves lack an "adequate" body of clinical evidence to substantiate their efficacy. Fortunately, they have not been found to be unsafe. Thus, those patients who are currently consuming these products and experiencing health benefits should not discontinue them. Based upon Commission E's findings, however, I must, at this time, recommend as a first choice for hawthorn, 160–900 mg native water-ethanol extract derived from leaf with flower to be divided into two or three doses daily.

Please be aware that—as with most herbs—clinical improvements may not be noted until the herb has been consistently consumed for at least four to six weeks.

Garlic (Allium sativum)

Garlic, a member of the lily family, has been used as an herbal medicine for over 5,000 years. Its salubrious effects span well beyond cardiovascular disease. Garlic has substantial antimicrobial benefits—combating bacteria, fungi, viruses, and even worms—along with its anticancer and immunity-enhancing values. Since garlic blocks the metabolism (breakdown) of insulin, it may possess glucose-lowering effects which can aid in the treatment of diabetic patients.

Garlic derives its healing properties from a sulfur-containing compound called "allicin." As anyone who cooks can attest, garlic is a pungent herb. Thus, it would be classified as an aromatic herb, deriving its benefit from the volatile oils of which allicin is a key component. Cooked garlic, however, is much less health-enhancing than raw garlic.

Obviously, if we wish to maintain our friends, we cannot consume raw garlic with impunity. Consequently, numerous companies have struggled to create a form of garlic which we can take without caus- ing bad breath and which also possesses clinical efficacy. Several good products now exist. When searching for a healthful product, find one which provides at least 10 mg of alliin, or a "total allicin po- tential" of 4,000 mcg daily. If you do take a garlic supplement, please don't stop cooking with this wonderful herb, as it not only enhances the flavor of food, but will also provide you with some additional health benefits.

Now that we know which forms of garlic are best, let's discover the cardiovascular advantages of this ancient herb. Garlic, like hawthorn, has found favor in the eyes of the German Commission E in the management of cardiovascular disease. Garlic is a powerful aid in the control of elevated cholesterol. Although a recent study failed to document the cholesterol lowering effect of this herb many studies have shown 10–15 percent decrements in total cholesterol and LDL levels from simple supplementing with garlic. Additionally, HDL levels have been noted to increase in many patients. Two of garlic's "anti-blood-clotting" effects—on platelets and fibrinogen— may also provide a significant advantage in the treatment of cardio- vascular patients. Garlic's antiplatelet effects, not too dissimilar to aspirin's, may help decrease the frequency of heart attacks and un- stable angina pectoris. Fibrinogen, a blood component promoting clotting, has been shown to be a potent risk factor for cardiac dis- ease. As garlic has been noted to counteract fibrinogen's effects, gar- lic can once again be understood as a valuable tool in the fight against atherosclerosis. In addition to its cholesterol-lowering and blood-thinning properties, garlic can decrease both systolic and di- astolic blood pressure in hypertensive patients.

With its strong antioxidant properties, garlic now joins the ranks of vitamins E and C in the war against free radical attack. Overall, garlic represents an herb which should be found routinely, not only in our kitchen cabinets but also on our supplement shelves.

Coleus Forskohii

Coleus, a member of the mint family, is an herb of the Ayurvedic tradition, whose active ingredient is "forskolin." On a cellular level, forskolin derives its activities by increasing levels of cyclic AMP (cAMP), which increase the heart's squeeze (inotropy), enhance arterial dilation, and promote platelet inhibition. From a cardiac perspective, coleus is useful in the treatment of high blood pressure, congestive heart failure, and angina pectoris. It works very well when given in conjunction with hawthorn. Coleus is an extremely safe herb and I have used it effectively in numerous patients as an aid in the treatment of hypertension. The recommended dosage is a standardized extract of 9 mg of forskolin taken two or three times daily.

Ginkgo Biloba

Although ginkgo biloba is the third most commonly consumed monosupplement in the United States, and although there are numerous studies documenting its efficacy in the treatment of a variety of disorders, I have, in certain circumstances (like the treatment of memory disorders), been disappointed with its outcomes. Ginkgo biloba extract is prepared from the leaves of a tree that can live up to 1,000 years. It is the oldest living tree species, dating back over 200 million years. The German Commission E has approved this ancient herb in three settings: (1) for the management of lower extremity pain caused by arterial blockage (called "intermittent claudication"), (2) for the treatment of memory deficits, as noted in patients with organic brain syndrome, and (3) in the treatment of vertigo and ringing in the ear (tinnitus). Because of a potential for allergic reactions, the Commission E recommends that ginkgolic acids be limited to less than 5 parts per million.

In my own patient population, I have found ginkgo beneficial in the treatment of lower extremity pain, vertigo, and ringing in the ears, but not in the management of patients suffering from memory disorders.

By telling you this, I do not wish to wipe away the world's literature supporting the use of ginkgo in patients with memory deficits. There are obviously enough individuals with memory disorders who have benefitted from ginkgo biloba to warrant its recommendation by the German Commission E. I relate my own experience simply as a means of underscoring the variety of possible outcomes in treating ailments not only with pharmaceutical drugs but also with herbal supplements. Additionally, if you, like millions of others, suffer from a faltering memory, please do not let my experience dissuade you from trying this potentially valuable herb. It is extremely safe. Only rarely do patients develop side effects such as headaches, flushing, or gastrointestinal discomfort. Because of ginkgo's antiplatelet effects, an extraordinarily unusual patient may experience an increased propensity to bleed. As long as you are observant, and under the watchful eye of a physician, you can safely enjoy many health benefits from this ancient remedy.

Once again, please remember to inform your physician before beginning any herbal supplement. This will enable him or her to help you monitor not only its side effects—however rare and slight they may be—but also its efficacy. Not only will you be helping yourself by being forthright with your physician, but you will be functioning as an invaluable teacher for your doctor. Your physician will be inspired to learn about herbal remedies, and he will also gain cognizance of the vast numbers of patients currently turning to herbs as a useful addition to their pharmacologic armamentarium.

Cayenne Pepper (Capsicum annuum)

Not only do chili and paprika (both members of the capsicum family) enhance culinary recipes, they also bestow cardiovascular benefits. In addition to their potent antioxidant attributes, studies show these fruits of capsicum to lower cholesterol and triglyceride levels. They have also been documented to diminish platelet aggregation and augment the blood's ability to break up clots. The vasodilating effects of cayenne may also help in the management of hypertension and congestive heart failure. Some of my patients who have complained of cold fingers and toes have enjoyed the warming effects of oral supplements of cayenne. You should be aware that the most clearly established benefit of cayenne, however, is in its topical form as a treatment for various painful skin disorders. Even the FDA has approved its use in the management of post-herpetic neuralgia (pain following an outbreak of herpes).

Gugulipid

An Ayurmedic herb extracted from the mukul myrrh tree, gugulipid has been used for years in the treatment of hypercholesterolemia. In fact, it has been an approved drug for treating high cholesterol in India since 1986. Studies documenting its benefits have demonstrated elevations of HDL and decrements of total cholesterol and LDL cholesterol. The recommended dosage of gugulipid is 25 mg of gugulsterone (its active compound) taken three times a day. Some studies have shown that this dosage will decrease total cholesterol and triglycerides by nearly 25 percent, very competitive reductions when compared with current pharmaceutical agents. Although I have not found gugulipid to be quite so potent in my clinical practice, I have had numerous patients achieve adequate benefit from the consumption of this herb. One of its major drawbacks, I feel, is its frequent dosing regimen. I am convinced that the need to take a drug three times a day limits its clinical utility. Perhaps those patients of mine who have not fared quite so well as studies suggest they should have been remiss in adhering to a thrice-daily dosage regimen. A once-a-day gugulipid preparation would be a wonderful formulation. Hopefully, as we continue to witness the burgeoning of the herbal marketplace, preparations such as once-daily gugulipid will become available.

Flavonoids

Although not a specific herb, but rather a class of compounds, flavonoids represent such a powerful plant resource for the management of cardiovascular disease that I have included them in the herbal section of this book. Bioflavonoids are plant pigments which are responsible for the colors of fruits and flowers. To date, over 4,000 flavonoid structures have been discovered.

The four major categories of flavonoids, each possessing cardiovascular benefits, are: proanthocianadins, green tea, citrus bioflavinoids, and quercetin. Although a variety of health-promoting benefits can be derived from these substances, I will describe only those that aid the cardiovascular system.

Proanthocianidins

Proanthocianidins, or procyanodolic oligomers (PCOs or OPCs) are the most popularized of the bioflavonoids. There has been a great deal of recent publicity surrounding these agents, as they represent the health-promoting elements in red wine. Supplements containing high levels of PCOs include grapeseed extract and pine bark extract. Some herbs, such as hawthorn, contain high quantities of proanthocianidins. From a cardiovascular perspective, proanthocianidins are endowed with two beneficial characteristics. First, they are very potent antioxidants. As we now know that free radicals are major threats to our cardiovascular health, antioxidants have become potent players in the quest for heart health. PCOs' second important cardiovascular benefit resides is their ability to protect collagen, a supporting structure throughout our bodies and a key element maintaining healthy blood vessels. By helping to maintain the structural integrity of collagen within our blood vessel walls, OPCs may lessen the likelihood of untoward cardiac events. A notable side benefit of their influence on collagen is their tendency to diminish the leakiness of blood vessels. Thus patients prone to the development of unsightly bruises can often be helped by the addition of grape seed extract to their supplement regimen.

Green Tea

Camellia sinensis is the source of both green and black tea. Green tea is formed when the freshly picked camellia leaves are promptly and lightly steamed—thereby inactivating enzymes which would otherwise have oxidized the leaves. Black tea results when light steaming is not performed. Black tea, therefore, is an oxidized version of green tea. During the oxidation process, myriad beneficial components of the leaves are lost. Thus, green tea possesses the greatest salutary rewards. Although its largest health advantage lies in green tea's ability to limit the development of cancer, it also possesses cardiovascular value. Green tea, a potent antioxidant, may help protect our blood vessels from the ravages of its oxidizing enemies.

Citrus Bioflavonoids

The most substantial benefit of the citrus bioflavonoids lies in their ability to impact favorably on blood vessels. These substances can help diminish the bruising and swelling that occur in the setting of sick blood vessels. As patients with diabetes mellitus may derive the greatest success from these substances, citrus bioflavonoids should become a routine component of their daily supplement schedule.

Quercetin

Quercetin is an extraordinarily active bioflavonoid that is present in many plant substances. Its dominant effect is as an anti-inflammatory agent, but as an inhibitor of aldose reductase—the enzyme responsible for the formation of potentially harmful sorbitol— quercetin may also possess potent protective properties for patients suffering from diabetes mellitus. One of the best natural sources of quercetin is onions, an herb closely related to garlic.

I am sure you can discern that, among all the bioflavonoids, the greatest cardiovascular benefits lie within the family of proanthocianidins. These are safe substances and probably should be a part of everyone's daily regimen; 30 to 50 mg represents a reasonable daily dose.

One final note with regard to the bioflavonoids: A citrus bioflavonoid found predominantly in grapefruit juice, named "naringin," has been documented to alter the blood levels of numerous pharmaceutical agents. Blood serum levels of calcium channel blockers, nonsteroidal anti-inflammatory drugs, Coumadin, and estrogens have been elevated by the concomitant consumption of large quantities of grapefruit juice. I, a grapefruit lover, reject admonitions to eliminate grapefruit from the diets of those who are taking prescription medications. Rather, I would suggest modest consumption. Grapefruit offers too many health benefits to be quickly and carelessly expunged from the diets of health-seeking Americans. Instead, I would recommend that those people who continue taking prescription medications while consuming grapefruit be monitored closely by their treating physicians. If the consequence of mounting levels of medications becomes evident, the dosage of these medicines can be diminished. Once again, it is imperative to inform your physician not only of your herbal and vitamin supplements, but also of your dietary inclinations.

Bilberry (Vaccinium myrtillus)

Bilberry, the European blueberry, is an herb which contains very potent bioflavonoid compounds known as anthocianocides. Although the German Commission E recognizes use of this herb only in the treatment of diarrhea and throat irritation, numerous other studies have documented its importance in the management of ocular disorders such as macular degeneration, diabetic retinopathy, and cataracts. Bilberry has also been proved beneficial in augmenting night vision. Interestingly, it was noted as effective in World War II when the British Royal Air Force used this herb on their fighter pilots. (The American Air Force used vitamin A.) I include bilberry in this cardiovascular section of herbology as it instills blood vessels with powerful, health-promoting effects. Arteries, capillaries, and veins all gain functional improvements when patients take bilberry extract. Undoubtedly, however, its most salutary effects rest in the realm of treating eye disease.

A 41-year-old colleague and friend of mine was stricken at the age of 37 with the premature onset of macular degeneration. As a result, he was forced to abandon his field of gastroenterology. He continues to work as an internist, but his failing vision precludes his performance of endoscopic procedures, the "bread and butter" of gastroenterology.

A few years ago, I tentatively approached my friend to share what I had learned regarding a natural approach to macular degeneration. He had been treated at Baskin Palmer, a superb world-renowned eye institute. Since he was being treated at such a "scientifically grounded" institution, I suspected that he would be taking some experimental drug to counteract his disease's progression. To my surprise and elation, when I discussed his possible use of various herbal supplements such as bilberry extract, he exclaimed that he was taking bilberry and others. His eye surgeon, it seems, had prescribed bilberry extract and high-dose antioxidants.

That a Baskin Palmer physician suggested bilberry extract tells me that, even within the most rigorously scientific circles, some experts are appreciating the significance of natural and herbal additives. By the way, my friend experienced a complete halt in the progression of his ailment. Now, several years after beginning his natural regimen, he is no worse off than he was at the outset. While there has been no regression of his disease, its lack of progression represents substantial support of bilberry's utility.

Although I am a cardiologist, I do not treat my patients in a vacuum. When they complain of noncardiovascular ailments, I feel compelled to try to relieve them of their suffering. Therefore, I have explored the use of herbs in the management of several noncardiac ailments. I will now share my experiences with several of these substances.

Anxiety and insomnia are prevalent problems for my patients. Kava (*Piper methysticum*), a member of the pepper family, is an excellent adjunct in managing anxiety *and* insomnia. Used in Pacific Island ceremonies for thousands of years, kava has also recently gained notice in the United States, especially as a means of reducing stress and easing the transition from wakefulness to sleep. Several trials have demonstrated its efficacy in anxiety reduction. Additionally, documentation also exists for higher doses being used as a soporific. I can attest to the benefits of kava, having tried both lower and higher dosage regimens. Lower doses do tend to result in a greater sense of ease and relaxation, while higher doses tend to strip away the day's stress, leading to a more profound and unencumbered sleep. In the treatment of anxiety take 25–75 mg of kava lactones three times daily. For sleep induction take approximately 200 mg of kava lactones at bedtime. Side effects are remote when limiting kava intake to the aforementioned dosages. Patients who take excessive amounts of kava, however, can develop side effects such as skin reactions, abnormalities in blood chemistries, and the development of bloody urine. Once again, these problems have not occurred when patients adhere to recommended dosages. Thus, the presence of side effects at high doses should not deter you from exploring the many benefits of kava (and other herbal supplements).

Valerian root (*Valerianae radix*), a malodorous herb, also possesses potent soporific effects. At a dose of 150–300 mg of the 0.8 percent valeric acid standardized extract, valerian can improve the quality of sleep in insomnia sufferers. If you can get beyond its foul smell, this herb will become a valuable addition to your pharmacopeia. On a personal note, I have not found this to be quite so effective as kava for the induction and maintenance of good sleep. I have cared for several patients, however, who can attest to its usefulness. As valerian is generally regarded as safe, it represents a reasonable choice for those patients who wish to avoid prescription drugs in managing their insomnia.

Saw palmetto berry (*Seranoa repens*) is an herb which has also received approval from the German Commission E, specifically in the management of urinary problems caused by nonmalignant prostate enlargement (benign prostatic hypertrophy or BPH). Through both its anti-androgenic and anti-estrogenic effects, saw palmetto is now known as an effective agent in managing BPH. Studies have demonstrated that within a four- to six-week span, nearly 90 percent of all patients experience significant improvements in the symptoms of benign prostatic hypertrophy when taking this herb.

In his book *The Healing Power of Herbs*, Michael T. Murray, N.D., compares the studies evaluating saw palmetto to those assessing Proscar, a pharmaceutical agent currently employed in managing BPH. He demonstrated that while 90 percent of all patients achieved prompt improvement in their symptoms when using saw palmetto extract, only 50 percent of those on Proscar documented improvement after taking their medication for one year. On a personal note, my father-in-law, a conservative but at times surprisingly open-minded cardiologist, has enjoyed a significant improvement in his symptoms of BPH through the effects of a supplement combining both saw palmetto and Pygeum. *Pygeum africanum*, an African evergreen, has also been shown to help alleviate the symptoms of BPH. Because of the synergism between saw palmetto and pygeum, several supplements now combine both herbs. Take a dose of 100–200 mg of a standardized pygeum extract and 320 mg of a standardized saw palmetto extract daily.

Feverfew (*Tanacetum parthenium*), a member of the sunflower family, has been shown to play a significant role in the prevention of migraine headaches. Migraines currently afflict 17 million Americans, to the tune of hundreds of millions of dollars annually (and a great deal of suffering). As current pharmaceutical agents possess potentially harmful side effects, a good natural remedy for this ailment would certainly be welcomed. Magnesium, a mineral, has also proved effective in managing migraines, with studies showing a nearly 80 percent amelioration of migraine symptoms. Feverfew, an herb, has similar benefits, with British studies revealing its importance in managing migraines. One trial demonstrated a diminution of frequency and intensity of migraine headaches in 70 percent of the patients studied. A double-blind study performed at the University of Nottingham demonstrated clear improvement in the frequency and severity of migraine headaches. Dosages required for adequate prophylaxis depend upon the content of parthenolide, this herb's active ingredient. It is suggested that 0.25–0.5 mg of parthenolide be taken daily in order to achieve the benefits of feverfew as documented in various studies.

For its part, we now know licorice (*Glycyrrhiza glabra*) is an effective aid in managing peptic ulcer disease when taken in its deglycyrrhizinated form—DGL or deglycyrrhizinated licorice. In its native form, licorice herb, can activate the effects of certain natural steroids: the glucocorticoids and mineral corticoids. Unfortunately, this steroid-augmenting effect can lead to elevations of blood pressure, retention of salt and water, and decreases in blood potassium levels. To enable people to derive the licorice's curative effects, while avoiding its potentially toxic effects, a deglycyrrhizinated form of licorice was developed (i.e., the glycycrrhiza has been removed). By chewing one to two tablets three or four times a day, many patients have been cured of their peptic ulcers. Accomplished without any significant side effects, this represents a great advance over many of the pharmaceutical agents employed in the management of this disorder. The problem with DGL, however, is that the tablets, which must be chewed, taste terrible! If, however, you suffer from peptic ulcer disease and are able tolerate the pungent licorice taste of DGL, ask your physician to help you use this herbal remedy in managing your condition. Both you and your doctor may be pleasantly surprised by its safe and salubrious impact.

Before departing this chapter, I wish to share a lesson I learned from my studies in nutritional herbology at Bastyr University. Herbs are wonderful, profoundly health-promoting natural substances which can be used in treating many health conditions. Their consumption, however, should not be limited to supplement form. By living with these herbs, incorporating them in your daily culinary creations, you can have fun in the kitchen while simultaneously supporting your health. By adding herbs such as ginger, cayenne, curry, onion, and garlic to your recipes, you will be taking advantage of nature's edible gifts. These tasteful delights can be savored through a continuous culinary exploration to reap their deepest rewards.

TABLE 25
Herbs Helpful in Managing Medical Ailments

Herb	Effect
Aromatic Herbs	
Clary sage Lemon Lavender Marjoram Thyme	• Lowers blood pressure.

TABLE 25 (Continued)
Herbs Helpful in Managing Medical Ailments

Herb	Effect
Valerian	• Causes sedation.
Bergamot	• Increases appetite. I had a patient with a decreased appetite who needed to eat, so his wife put some bergamot on a towel and had him hold it over his face. His appetite returned almost immediately.
Peppermint	• Eases headaches. • Improves digestion.
Ylang/ylang Orange Patchouli	• Causes relaxation.

Astringent Herbs

White willow bark	• Pain killer or analgesic. Salicylates, the active compounds in aspirin, come from this plant. White willow bark is a safer painkiller than aspirin, because it contains mucilage that protects the stomach, which aspirin can damage.

Bitter Herbs

Cascara sagrada bark Sarsaparilla root	• Acts as a laxative. • Useful for skin diseases (such as psoriasis), arthritis, and as a diuretic.

Mucilaginous Herbs

Slippery elm	• Used to treat sore throat (can swallow capsule or break them open) or upset stomach.
Aloe leaf	• Acts as a laxative and demulcent.

Nutritive Herbs

Asparagus root	• Contains vitamin A, vitamin B, folic acid, copper, magnesium, and potassium.
Spirulina algae	• Contains protein, chromium, iron, manganese, zinc, and B_1, B_2, B_3.
Rose hips fruit	• During World War II, Europeans discovered that rose hips were the best source of vitamin C, although some of the vitamin is loss in processing. Rose hips also contains calcium and vitamins A, E, B_1, B_2.

To Sweat or Not to Sweat—It Is No Longer a Question

Your alarm rings. It's 6:00 A.M., and you have to get to the gym before heading off to work. You rub your eyes, fall out of bed, get yourself ready, and depart. Driving, you ask yourself whether an extra hour of sleep might have been better for you than the exercise you are about to endure. As you step on the treadmill and begin your 3–5-minute warm-up, you are still questioning the importance of this early-morning torment. By the time you are into your weight-lifting regimen, however, you're invigorated, empowered and very wide awake. You've already begun to answer your own question—yes, it is absolutely worth the trouble it takes to maintain a regular exercise regimen.

I have always been active and fairly fit. In high school, I played tennis and swam. In college, I studied the martial arts, ultimately achieving a black belt in Tae Kwon Do. During those years, I exercised two, sometimes even three, hours a day. When I began medical school, however, things changed. I no longer allotted time in my schedule for exercise. Exercise became a burden rather than a pleasure. By the time I finished my residency and fellowship training programs, I was clearly out of shape. When I began my private practice in cardiology, things got no better. In fact, I became more and more sedentary. With the births of my three children, my responsibilities and obligations grew. To exercise would mean to spend less time with my growing family. Therefore, I continued to sacrifice my own physical and mental well-being for the presumed benefit of my loved ones.

A few years ago, I was blessed with the revelation that the sacrifice of my own physical and mental health was, in fact, not beneficial to my children. I realized that a greater gift to them would be to become a father who was active both physically and mentally and, therefore, had a greater chance of living a longer, healthier, and more productive life.

I forged my commitment to exercise, went to my local gym, and hooked up with a wonderful personal, trainer, Shaun O'Hare. Shaun, having a masters degree in exercise physiology, not only trained me to improve my physical fitness, but also taught me much of the science behind my exercises.

Initially, I was extremely reluctant to include resistance training, or weight lifting, in my exercise regimen—reluctant and a bit embarrassed. I had never been a weight lifter and looked it! With time, however, I learned the many health benefits of resistance training. Not only did I shed fat and weight with exercise, but I also began to feel much more energized. I began to understand that waking up early to go to the gym deprived me of sleep but nevertheless infused me with energy. In this chapter, I will describe the many health benefits of exercise. So that you may develop a deeper understanding of what you're doing when you sweat in the gym, I will review and define pertinent exercise terminology.

Although they may seem self-explanatory, the four principles of exercise include: *intensity*, which refers to the difficulty of a particular type of training; *frequency*, which refers to how often one trains; *mode*, signifying the type of exercise chosen; and the *duration*, implying the total time of exercise.

There are three major modes of exercise: aerobic (or cardiovascular), anaerobic (now often called "resistance training"), and flexibility training.

Aerobic Training

To achieve cardiovascular benefits, one must begin an aerobic training program. This type of exercise employs large muscle groups for prolonged periods of time. One must have the appropriate intensity, frequency, mode, and duration of exercise to achieve cardiovascular benefits—just any exercise program will not accomplish this goal.

With regard to intensity, it has been found that exercising at about 70 percent of your maximal predicted heart rate is required to ensure good cardiovascular effects. Determining one's maximum heart rate is very easy. A simplified equation is as follows: maximum predicted heart rate = 220 minus your age. For example, a 40-year-old has a maximum predicted heart rate of 220 minus 40 or 180; 70 percent of 180 is 126. Therefore, this 40-year-old must exercise at a steady heart rate of approximately 126 beats per minute in order to achieve the full cardiovascular benefits that can be derived from aerobic training.

To attain optimal benefits from training, one must perform aerobic exercise at least three times a week. The A-Strand study, which looked at Scandinavian cross-country skiers, was the trial that established the basis for recommending three training sessions per week. In this study, one or two sessions a week did not result in a significant training effect. This, of course, does not mean that one should limit oneself to three sessions a week. In fact, some studies have shown that, by exercising four or five times a week, improved weight loss is a near certainty.

With regard to the mode of aerobic training, a variety of exercises are beneficial: walking, jogging, running, bicycling, stair climbing, cross-country skiing, and performing land and water aerobics are a few of the best. In deciding which form of exercise to choose, pick a suitable one. In other words, find something you enjoy doing. If you hate running, don't run. If swimming bothers your ears and eyes, don't swim. There is a wide enough range of choices available to keep almost anyone happy.

Remember, too, that you do not have to stick to one form of aerobic training. Varying your exercise will keep it interesting and exciting and thus increase the likelihood that you will continue your exercise regimen.

Now that you know *how* to engage in an aerobic training regimen, you might ask yourself *why* you must do this. There are countless benefits to aerobic exercise. For example, both systolic and diastolic blood pressure usually decrease with exercise. As you know, decreasing one's blood pressure translates into a fall in the risk of future heart attacks, strokes, and kidney damage. When performing aerobic training, HDL increases while LDL and triglycerides decrease. These lipid advantages also result in a drop in the risk of cardiovascular disease.

During training, there is also a *direct* impact on the heart muscle it-self. An exerciser's heart can become larger, stronger, and more efficient. Each beat of the heart can deliver more blood, oxygen, and nutrients to the brain, muscles, and other vital organs. Even blood vessels themselves change in the setting of aerobic training. Vessels become healthier and stronger while capillaries increase in number, thus improving the blood supply to muscle fibers and other tissues. This endows the exerciser with the ability to work longer and recover faster than an untrained individual.

Lung function is also improved with aerobic training. Oxygen transport and carbon dioxide removal are made more efficient through exercise. Both the resting heart rate and the heart rate needed to sustain a strenuous activity are decreased in trained individuals. This translates into less oxygen consumption by the heart. In patients with documented coronary disease, exercise training will thus enable them to perform greater activity with less angina.

Aerobic exercise has also been demonstrated to decrease the emergence of coronary heart disease. A study of British civil servants demonstrated that those who exercised had a significantly lower incidence of heart disease than those who were sedentary. This benefit was also documented in studies of San Francisco dockworkers and Harvard University alumni.

In addition to the physical effects of exercise, there are also psychological benefits. Studies have shown that regular exercise can at times be as effective as psychotherapy in the treatment of clinical depression. It has also been shown that anxiety levels are decreased in people engaged in regular training programs. If you are a nonexerciser, I hope you are beginning to sense the value of exercise.

Resistance or Weight Training

There are two fundamental goals in weight training: to improve *strength* and *endurance*. Strength can be defined as the momentary force generated by a muscle or muscle group. Muscular endurance is defined as the ability of a muscle or muscle group to generate force for a prolonged period of time. Each of these functions has its benefits and, therefore, must be developed during weight training. You can achieve improvements in muscle strength and endurance by utilizing the principle of progressive overload. Experiencing an overload or excessive weight will cause a muscle to increase in strength, endurance, and metabolic rate. Of course, the type of overload you use in resistance training will determine the relative benefits to your strength or endurance. When assessing resistance training we again utilize the already familiar principles of intensity, frequency, duration, and mode.

In weight training, intensity is measured by the amount of weight lifted. (In aerobic training, the maximum heart rate is used to determine the intensity of exercise.) During resistance training, the one repetition maximum (one RM) is the basis for determining the intensity of an individual exercise. The one repetition maximum represents the maximum amount of weight an individual can lift one time for a given exercise. In order to achieve maximum *strength* gains, set your exercise intensity at 80–90 percent of the one repetition maximum. You should lift this particular weight 3–8 times, performing 3–8 "repetitions per set." If muscular *endurance* rather than strength improvement is your goal, lower your exercise intensity to 60–80 percent of the one repetition maximum. In addition to lifting lighter weights, you will also perform more repetitions, with an advisable range of 8–15.

As is the case with most aspects of life, balance is essential in realizing "healthful" resistance training. You can balance strength and endurance gains through a weight training program which consists of exercising at an intensity of 70–80 percent of the one RM, with 10–12 repetitions per set. When just beginning a resistance training program, perform only 1 or 2 sets at a time. Later, after six to eight weeks, you can increase the number of sets.

The frequency and duration of a weight training program are dependent upon the intensity of the exercises. As the intensity increases, the frequency and duration can decrease; while at lower intensity, frequency and duration should increase. A schedule of two to three exercise sessions a week, each lasting thirty minutes to one hour, is appropriate for individuals embarking upon a weight-training routine. It must be remembered, though, that muscles should be allowed to recover completely (all pain must dissipate) before restressing them with additional weight training.

There are two common modes of resistance training: isometric and isotonic. Isometric exercise refers to the contraction of a muscle in the absence of movement. Examples of this kind of exercise are pushing against a wall, and "making a muscle." Although strength can be increased with isometric exercise, its drawbacks limit its applicability. Not only is it difficult to measure success with isometric exercise, but the absence of motion with this form of training restricts any benefit to a very limited area of the muscle.

Isotonic training, on the other hand, refers to muscle contraction with movement through a full range of motion. This is currently the most popular and effective method of weight training. Free weights and weight machines are the workhorses of isotonic resistance training. While it is difficult to measure progress when using isometric techniques, isotonic exercise will enable you to reap the benefits of positive reinforcement as you increase the weight loads you can lift with greater ease.

There is a common misconception (which I also used to believe) that weight-training benefits are limited to aesthetic improvements. This could not be further from the truth. Resistance training increases the exerciser's metabolism, resulting in a greater capacity to burn fat and thus reduce total body fat. Therefore, not only does the weight lifter look better, but he or she is, in fact, healthier. An increase in lean muscle tissue parallels a decrease in total body fat. Weight training also reduces the risk of orthopedic and muscular injuries, and because it produces an increase in bone density, it lowers the risk of osteoporosis. Some studies have also suggested that diabetics achieve the added benefit of stabilizing blood sugar levels when performing weight training. Additionally, any weight lifter can tell you that overall stress is decreased through enhanced physical activity.

As in the case with aerobic training, we must not forget that overall quality of life improves with weight training. As we enhance our self-confidence and self-esteem, we also reduce our anxiety and depression. Nor are the benefits of weight training confined to the young and healthy. Older people can dramatically enhance their lives by beginning a resistance training program. In fact, the elderly can increase muscle mass just as readily as their younger counterparts. Research has also shown that older individuals who begin resistance training are usually stronger, healthier, and less depressed than older people who don't exercise at all. So it's truly never too late to begin a properly supervised weight-lifting program.

Flexibility

The most misunderstood and neglected element of exercise is flexibility enhancement. Even exercise fanatics are often remiss when it comes to flexibility training. The problem with flexibility is that its enhancement does not result in any immediate visible improvements. Unless you are a yogi, gymnast, or martial artist you rarely have the opportunity to demonstrate improvements in flexibility during routine daily physical activity. Unfortunately, however, the absence of flexibility training predisposes individuals to the development of musculoskeletal problems. For example, low back pain, which afflicts millions of Americans, usually results from a musculoskeletal disorder. Improvements in hamstring and low back range of motion will often relieve the vast majority of low back pain problems. If people practiced flexibility techniques on a regular basis, they would be much less prone to develop back problems and other musculoskeletal disorders in the first place.

During my years of performing Tae Kwon Do flexibility training was an integral part of my daily routine. I spent literally fifteen to thirty minutes a day stretching in order to protect my muscles from the potential tears and strains which could result from such a vigorous and ballistic form of exercise. Only once during my years of martial arts training did I injure a muscle, and that was when I foolishly neglected to stretch before my workout.

To enhance flexibility, there are three common stretching techniques: static, ballistic, and proprioceptive neuromuscular facilitation (PNF). Static stretching is the most commonly employed technique and for the majority of people represents the best way to achieve good flexibility. During this activity, one slowly stretches his muscle toward the end of a range of motion, the stretch is held for at least ten seconds, and minimal pain should be experienced. You will be pleasantly surprised to see how rapidly you can achieve improvement when performing static stretching on a regular basis.

Ballistic, or dynamic stretching, employs fast, jerky muscle movements as one attempts to force a muscle beyond the point of easy stretching. This form of flexibility training was more prevalent ten to twenty years ago, but has since been found to result in muscle soreness and even muscle tears. I, therefore, do not advocate the use of ballistic flexibility training.

Proprioceptive neuromuscular facilitation (PNF) is a more complex form of stretching which involves isometric contraction of muscle groups, followed by a relaxed static stretching of the muscles. Although this form of stretching is beneficial, it is somewhat more complicated to perform and only people who are more proficient in flexibility training should use it. For those of you who are weight trainers and suffer from the frequent delayed-onset muscle soreness (DOMS), you should know that flexibility training provides not only the aforementioned benefits but also helps limit this form of soreness by promoting the removal of waste products and the transport of nutrient-rich blood to exercising muscles. Although it is unusual to witness weight lifters stretching out after they exercise, those who are "in the know" understand its benefits and can be seen stretching after each set.

I hope you are now convinced that exercise is not merely a means of improving your appearance. Regular exercise—employing aerobic, resistance, and flexibility training—will endow you with important physical, emotional, and psychological benefits. Yes, you will look better, but you will also feel better and live longer after you get hooked on exercise.

One final word of advice: Have a certified trainer help you through the first several months of your new exercise program. This will be money well spent, as it will enable you to reap the rewards of exercise without suffering the possible injuries which may result from unsupervised training.

CHAPTER 14

You Needn't Be a Yogi to Be Relaxed

The existence of stress is an ineluctable element of life. Stress surrounds us. Without warning, it often pierces our very being, bringing us to our emotional knees, at times crippling us with despair. The old adage stating that life's only constants are death and taxes should probably be restated as "life's only constant is stress." Death and taxes clearly fall under the aegis of stress.

Not all stress is bad, however. In fact, when viewing our evolution, we can certainly understand the protective physiologic elements of the stress response. Sudden or acute stress evokes a stimulation of the sympathetic nervous system. Epinephrine and norepinephrine (adrenaline) are released from nerves and the adrenal glands. These surging levels of adrenaline result in rising blood pressure, heart rate, heart muscle contractility, air exchange, and an increased delivery of blood to muscles. Like a supercharged superhero, the stress-altered human animal is readied for battle.

In the days of our remote ancestors, this altered state surely saved lives. Attacked by a wild beast, for example, the stress-enhanced human being was better able either to enter battle or flee the situation. This "fight or flight" response enables human beings to react to danger physically with boosted speed, strength, and tenacity. Thus, in the context of a "real" life-or-death event, our physiologic response to stress is quite a gift.

Within our "civilized" world, however, stress has taken on maleficent characteristics. And in that regard, it is our maladaptive response to stress that presently plagues us. For example, when we experience a stress-related physical response to a nonphysical threat, we have responded inappropriately. Repeated erroneous rousing of the fight or flight response can result in chronic physical ailments such as hypertension, high cholesterol, heart attacks, increased blood clotting, and strokes. To perceive the magnitude of this problem, let's view a day in the life of a typical American woman.

We'll start in the middle of the night. Two A.M.: The tiny hands of your youngest child tap your sleeping shoulder to notify you of the day's first "fire" that you alone can extinguish. Exhausted, you fall from your bed, shuffle to your daughter's room, and change the bedding that has been soaked by an untimely nighttime stream. You change her pajamas and convince her to sleep the remainder of the night in her own bed. Although you try to be soft and comforting, you can't help feeling angry that your shattered slumber will certainly leave you weakened in your quest to meet the next day's demands. Extra adrenaline has already seeped into places where it does not belong. You are lucky, though, and you fall back to sleep.

Six A.M.: Alarms buzz. It's time to face the day. You shower and dress while your children sleepily enter your room to expound their litany of reasons why they shouldn't go to school. You struggle with them to shower, eat breakfast, brush their teeth, turn the TV off, and buckle their seat belts so that they can get to school on time. It's going to be close, so you pray that the traffic light gods will be smiling on you. Unfortunately, you neglected to pay due homage to the incredibly-annoying-driver-in-front-of-you god, and you are cursed. The right lane is appropriately slow but directly in front of you in the "fast" left lane drives a casually cruising individual who is clearly independently wealthy, since he certainly cannot be driving to work. Your blood begins to boil. Again, you are eliciting the fight or flight response. With each glance at the clock, epinephrine pumps through your body. Your blood pressure rises, your heart pounds heavily in your chest and races as you search for an escape route to skirt your oblivious foe. It is only 8:00 A.M. and already your body has been barraged by an unnecessary hormonal attack. No tigers have threatened your life. You have not had to run from an approaching tidal wave. No physical circumstances have threatened you, and yet your body has already readied itself for several battles.

You make it to school on time (barely), hug and kiss your kids, and travel to work. Yes, in addition to raising children, you are also employed. You remind yourself that work enables you to remain connected to the adult world, while simultaneously helping meet the family's burgeoning budgetary demands. You race through the day, knowing that school pickup is at 3:15. Instead of pacing yourself at work, you pack eight hours into six, neglecting breaks and healthful lunches. Now you have activated not only the sympathetic nervous system, but also the hypothalamic-pituitary-adrenal-cortical axis, thereby increasing your blood levels of cortisol. This inappropriate elevation of cortisol, which can become chronic, will lead to higher blood glucose levels, weight gain (from fat), increased LDL cholesterol, decreased sexual function, and a diminution in body repair mechanisms. Not good! You meet your children at school so you may shuttle them to their diverse and distant after-school activities. Somehow you find time to go grocery shopping, make dinner, and clean the house.

After dinner, you juggle your children's homework needs. Finally, you ready them all for bed. Books are read, stories told; by 9:00 P.M., they are asleep. Now it is your time. You can lie back, kick up your heels, and enjoy a good book and a cup of tea. As you settle in, you hear a faint hallucination. No, there it is again. This time a little louder—it is real: "Honey, can you scratch my back?" Your day is complete. And this was a day devoid of crisis, casualty, or real hardship.

Stress is life. Life is stress. The issue is how to live with stress—which is unavoidable—and yet train your body to overcome its primitively programmed and potentially harmful responses to stress. Although all of us live with stress, some of us cope better than others.

The creation of coping strategies can endow individuals with stress-protective shields. These escutcheons are not external, however. They represent internal alterations in our behavior patterns which enable us to deflect stressful circumstances and limit their impact on our bodies. By creating these protective shields, we will not necessarily diminish the frequency of stressful insults, but rather we will alter our own perception of and reaction to these events.

Our Reactions to Stress

There is a wide range of psychological risk factors that have been noted to predispose patients to developing heart disease. They include Type A behavior pattern, social isolation or lack of social support, anger and hostility, depression, anxiety, and even simply worrying.

Let's first assess the *Type A behavior pattern*. In the 1950s, two cardiologists from San Francisco, Meyer Friedman and Ray Rosenman, coined the term "Type A behavior pattern" (TABP). A typical individual suffering from TABP can be recognized by a variety of symptoms and signs. Typically an insecure individual, he possesses inadequate self-esteem. He often has an intense sense of time urgency and experiences hyperaggressive and free-floating hostility. He attempts to perform more than one task at a time, often dislikes waiting in lines, demonstrates fetishistic punctuality, and (because it is too "relaxing") rarely is found daydreaming. You can recognize this individual by his chronic facial tension, tense posture, and rapid speech. He often hastens the speech of others saying "uh-huh, uh-huh." A type A individual will commonly lose his temper while driving. He is usually extremely irritable and often suffers from profound intramarital tensions. Type A individuals are typically insomniacs, as a consequence of their extreme anxiety and free-floating anger. These individuals have been assessed in a variety of studies including the Western Collaborative Group Study, The Framingham Heart Study, and the MRFIT. In fact, a meta-analysis of 83 trials revealed that the risk of coronary heart disease is doubled in patients with type A behavior patterns.

It has recently been asserted that anger and hostility probably represent the single most malignant component of type A behavior patterns. Anger has even been demonstrated to trigger myocardial infarctions. A 1992 "anger recall" study demonstrated a decrease in our heart muscle's function that was associated with hostile sentiments. In 1993, a study of patients undergoing cardiac catheterizations showed that anger can result in vasoconstriction (tightening of our blood vessels).

A number of years ago, I was an impotent witness to the devastating power of *anger*. At the time, I was caring for a 75-year-old woman who required a coronary artery bypass surgery. The patient had a strong heart muscle, yet she suffered from severe blockages in all three blood vessels feeding her heart. Since she endured intractable angina, she reluctantly agreed to undergo a life-saving bypass operation. She had struggled fiercely to avoid this operation, but her two daughters convinced her of its necessity. In a sense, they "guilted" her into this procedure by telling her that she would be acting selfishly and unfairly by dying without making every attempt to prolong her own life. The patient went through the operation without a hitch.

The day after surgery, I visited her on my morning rounds. She was awake, alert, and very responsive. She was also furious. In pain, she cursed the fact that her daughters had made her endure this operation. She proclaimed that she wanted to die. I sat with her for a long while, pleading with her to have a more positive attitude and imploring her to drop her death wish. She was intransigent. I left her bedside and summoned her two daughters. Sitting with these young women, I informed them that their mother's threats should be taken extremely seriously. Believing in the power of the mind's influence over the body, I warned them that their mother could die if she continued to experience her anger-motivated desideratum.

Her daughters pleaded with her, yet their exchange was angry. Their mother continued along her unyielding path. When her daughters left, I remained frightened. Unfortunately, my fears were justified. Two hours later, my patient experienced ventricular fibrillation, a typically lethal heart rhythm disturbance. Since she was in the intensive care unit, all appropriate measures were taken immediately to try to terminate this arrhythmia. All efforts failed. She died in the absence of a sound medical (or physical) explanation. My belief is that our patient committed suicide. Anger was her weapon.

Like many researchers involved in the study of psychological risk factors for heart disease, I believe that anger represents the dominant component of the type A behavior pattern which is responsible for the development of coronary heart disease.

It is important to note that by acknowledging our emotions' impact upon our bodies, we understand that our minds can, in fact, either willfully or unwillfully control our physical beings. Our patient clearly killed herself with a thought; and if people can do something as dramatic and devastating as that, then they can undoubtedly influence other aspects of their physical state as well.

The new discipline of psychoneuroimmunology (PNI) addresses this very phenomenon. PNI investigates pathways and relationships between the mind and the body. This burgeoning field is, in truth, the framework within which a whole new world of science and healing will evolve. It is my futuristic belief that, over the next ten to twenty years, a medical metamorphosis will occur in which our minds will become our greatest allies in the quest for health.

As a medical student I was taught that *stress* played no role in the development of heart attacks, yet studies have demonstrated that nearly 50 percent of all heart attacks are preceded by a strong emotional stressor. Other studies have demonstrated that 50 percent of all patients with coronary disease experience "silent ischemia" under stressful circumstances. We also know that many episodes of sudden cardiac death are precipitated by stressful episodes. This may be due to the fact that psychological stress can diminish the threshold for ventricular fibrillation, a frequently fatal rhythm disturbance like the one which killed our angry patient. Serum lipids, critical culprits in the creation of coronary disease, seem to peak at times of stress. For example, accountants experience their highest serum lipid levels on April 15th (their—and our—day of reckoning). Similarly, medical students have their highest serum lipids during final examinations. Stress thus alters many of our bodies' components in a potentially damaging and frequently silent fashion.

Social isolation has also been noted to represent a significant psychological stress which can predispose an individual to the development of coronary artery disease. In some studies, lack of significant social support has been found to be as great a risk factor as cigarette smoking. For example, unmarried patients demonstrate a higher mortality rate after myocardial infarctions than married patients. Thus some sort of support group can be extremely helpful in managing coronary artery disease patients. Clinical depression has also been found to predispose patients to developing untoward cardiovascular events. In fact, *depression* is one of the best predictors of adverse events after acute myocardial infarctions.

It is my ardent hope that by acknowledging our own role in the genesis of heart disease (and other physical ailments), we will all try to find ways to improve our potentially life-saving coping mechanisms.

Stress Reduction Techniques

There are two distinct approaches to achieving a resolution of stress. The simplest styles aim to provide rapid but transient relief of stressful circumstances. The other, more comprehensive school of relaxation promotion seeks to instill more permanent alterations in an individual's approach to life. These latter techniques typically begin in the setting of stress-free moments, and then move on to investigate those personal and individual behaviors which either facilitate or create internal stress. These techniques enable individuals to identify self-defeating habitual tendencies. People are made aware of the need to assume responsibility for their own actions. An enhancement of awareness permits patients to observe themselves and the world in a new light—a light which clarifies maladaptive responses to events and interpersonal relations.

Let us begin our scan of stress-reduction techniques with the simplest of approaches: diaphragmatic breathing. This elementary technique effectively decreases the stress of the moment. To perform diaphragmatic breathing, you must relax your belly. You then inhale deeply, expanding your belly before the expansion of your chest. Exhalation draws the belly gently in, allowing for deep and complete elimination of air "toxins." Diaphragmatic breathing is an infant's natural form of respiration. This, like many other youthful gifts, is usually lost from the repertoire of adults. You can perform this type of breathing at any time, and if you do it now, you will note a sudden soothing sense of peace circulating throughout your being.

Humor is another form of stress relief that can be performed in the moment. In Alan Klein's book *The Healing Power of Humor*, he describes numerous techniques for "getting through loss, setbacks, upsets, disappointments, difficulties, trials, tribulations and all that not so funny stuff." He describes vividly how humor helped him deal with the untimely death of his beloved wife. On a physical basis, humor has been shown to affect most physiologic systems of the human body. For example, heart rate and blood pressure tend to rise and then fall with a good guffaw. Laughter as a cardiovascular exercise has been described as being nine times as effective as the experience of difficult rowing.

Music is a gift that can also be used as a stress reduction tool, eliciting physiologic changes which enhance relaxation. Aromatherapy, like music and the other aforementioned techniques, can also be used to diminish stress "in the moment."

For example, consider this scenario. You are returning home from an extraordinarily stress-filled day at the office. Your mind spills over with thoughts of the day—conflicts, issues, unresolved questions. You enter your house, hanging your head low, yearning for the moment when you can lie down in silence and shut the world out. As you walk in, though, you are struck by an overwhelming sensation. Into your nostrils flows the aroma of freshly baked cookies, and peace permeates you. You are transported to your childhood when you would return home from school to sit quietly at the kitchen table while your mother presented you with freshly baked cookies and a large glass of whole milk. Your olfactory sense, an ancient but powerful part of your brain, has instantly facilitated your transport from present to past, and this experience leaves you cleansed of your day's quandaries.

I am not, of course, advocating using food as a stress-reduction tool, but pointing out that a simple smell has the power to purge us of burdensome emotions. This power can be harnessed through the use of aromatherapy. Ylang-ylang, patchouli, and lavender are just a few of the scents imbued with calming properties. Once again, aromatherapy, like previously mentioned techniques, represents a momentary solution to the problem of stress. To achieve a more profound and permanent transformation, an individual must explore and study other more comprehensive stress-reduction techniques.

Transcendental Meditation and the Relaxation Response

Transcendental meditation was introduced into the United States in 1959 by Maharishi Mahesh Yogi of India. This form of meditation, sometimes abbreviated as "TM," was extracted from yoga traditions and simplified to become more accessible to the average American. Basically, the technique is as follows: A trained instructor provides a secret word, sound, or phrase termed a "mantra." While sitting comfortably, the meditator mentally repeats his mantra. This repetition is meant to prevent distracting thoughts. When other thoughts enter their minds, the meditators discard them passively, without inner hostility, and then return their attention to the mantra. It's advised to meditate for twenty minutes in the morning before breakfast and again for twenty minutes in the evening before dinner.

Studies have demonstrated that this form of meditation can have profound physical effects. Oxygen consumption is lowered, the metabolic rate is diminished, and alpha waves—the type of brain waves prominent during times of peaceful relaxation—abound during transcendental meditation. Elevated blood pressure has also been found to fall during and after periods of TM.

Out of transcendental meditation grew Herbert Benson's development of the "relaxation response." Herbert Benson, M.D., a Harvard professor, studied individuals who practiced transcendental meditation techniques. Over the years, he discovered a variety of beneficial physical and emotional consequences from TM, and from his studies, he developed the relaxation response.

To evoke the relaxation response, Dr. Benson suggests that one sits quietly in a comfortable position with his or her eyes closed. The individual then attempts to relax all of the muscles, beginning at the feet and progressing up to the face. Breathing is performed through the nose, and Dr. Benson suggests that as one breathes in and out, he or she silently repeats the word "one," over and over again. As with TM, this practice should be performed at least twenty minutes daily. Dr. Benson advises us not to elicit the relaxation response within two hours of a meal, since it may interfere with the digestive process.

In his book *The Relaxation Response,* Dr. Benson details the many physiological advantages of his stress reduction technique. Blood pressure is lowered, epinephrine/norepinephrine levels are diminished, alpha waves are increased, and oxygen consumption is diminished, similar to the effects produced by TM. The relaxation response results from a profound stimulation of the parasympathetic nervous system. This is in direct opposition to the fight or flight response, during which the sympathetic nervous system dominates. Dr. Benson believes that repeated evocation of the relaxation response will limit the daily and unhealthful occurrence of the fight or flight response.

Mindfulness-Based Stress Reduction (MBSR) and Other Stress Reduction Techniques

This mode of stress reduction incorporates a "mindful meditation" that helps you develop awareness and observation. The practitioner experiences an inner perception of what the mind is thinking and the body feeling. During this form of meditation, the meditator focuses on breathing, slowly expanding the field of awareness to perceive all sense experiences. As feelings flow in and out of the practitioner, he or she simply observes them. This experience reminds me of a poem by William Blake which goes as follows: "He who tries to catch a joy/does that winged thing destroy,/but he who kisses it as it flies,/lives in eternity's sunrise."

During this peaceful, wordless internal dialogue, the only true focus of concentration is on breathing, and the meditator will develop a deeper consciousness of his or her relationship to the world. As he or she learns and grows, he or she will develop greater coping mechanisms, enabling him or her to face stressful circumstances without succumbing to previously maladaptive behavior patterns.

Along with mindfulness-based meditation, transcendental meditation, and the relaxation response, several other techniques are available. The body scan, progressive muscle relaxation, and visualization techniques are often helpful at eliminating stress by training one's body to become relaxed.

In the body scan, practitioners concentrate on individual components of their bodies, for instance, beginning at a toe and then moving all the way to the top of the head. Just as in the case of meditation techniques, patients are advised to be completely nonjudgmental. Thus, if they shift their focus of attention, they are instructed not to berate themselves, but rather to refocus their attention on a given body part.

During progressive muscle relaxation, as each body part is encountered, it is first tensed and then relaxed, eliciting a more thorough and complete sense of relaxation.

During visualization, an individual creates an image of serenity, whether it be lying at the beach or walking along pristine forest paths. All of these modalities permit practitioners to experience relaxation while also training their bodies and minds to live in greater peace and harmony.

Freeze frame, a stress reduction technique developed by a company called Heart-Math, enables practitioners to enjoy not only an enhanced state of self-awareness, but also a coping tool that can be used "in the moment" to alleviate stress. This practice, like other successful techniques, begins with awareness, specifically of a stressful feeling. Once a person grows conscious of an unpleasant feeling (a very important accomplishment in and of itself), he or she "takes a time out" or "freeze frames" and shifts his or her focus inward, literally to the area of the heart. He or she then recalls a prior warm, wonderful feeling and attempts to reexperience it. After this emotion of elation has literally washed through the practitioner, he or she "asks" the heart for advice and direction with regard to the current stress. Although this technique may at first glance appear contrived, it can, in fact, be extremely powerful and effective. I have tried it, and it works.

As a cardiologist, I find a special allure in freeze frame, as it acknowledges our heart's unique role not only as a vital organ and the seat of our emotions, but also as a profound and unrecognized source of intelligence. The heart is a complex and multifaceted organ, and freeze frame takes full advantage of its capabilities. What freeze frame appears to lack in spirituality, it makes up for in practicality. For people who cannot "get into" meditation, freeze frame offers an excellent alternative.

Two other relaxation techniques very well worth mentioning are yoga and T'ai Chi Chuan. Both of these styles incorporate exercise into the stress-reduction process. Yoga utilizes specific postures which the participant assumes with a slow deliberate awareness. These postures, in conjunction with highly developed breathing techniques, represent gentle forms of exercise which greatly reduce stress. Dr. Dean Ornish's successful program causing regression of coronary disease utilized yoga as its stress-reduction technique.

T'ai Chi Chuan (T'ai Chi) is an ancient art created from a unification of three powerful forces—Taoist thought, traditional Chinese medicine, and proven martial arts techniques. This "soft" martial art is not only one of the most powerful fighting tools, but also a way of life, blending yin and yang opposites into a balanced and healthy whole. Committed devotion to either T'ai Chi Chuan or yoga will strengthen not only the body, but the mind as well.

For all seekers of enhanced spirituality, in conjunction with healthier minds and bodies, I ardently advocate the study of either T'ai Chi Chuan or yoga.

I must emphasize that, although we are united in humanity, we are all individuals possessing idiosyncratic likes and dislikes. I could, therefore, never claim that one relaxation technique is better than another. My strong suggestion, however, is that everyone become aware of the need for introspection and emotional development. We all need to pursue some sort of stress reduction. I implore us all to love ourselves, and in so doing heal our minds as well as our bodies.

The Future of
Integrative Heart Care

Human beings are a species of individuals. Each of us is unique, possessing his or her own distinct fingerprints and retinal arteries. Metaphorically, therefore, each of us feels and sees the world uniquely. This individuality is both a blessing and a curse. Although it is an essential element of creativity, it also often represents a stumbling block to the reconciliation of conflicts. As human beings continue to evolve, I believe we will someday achieve a state of being in which, as individuals, we feel our human connectedness. I can visualize a day when we are all connected in the human struggle and the human glory. Unfortunately, we have not yet achieved this lofty state. Instead, individuals yearning for a greater connectedness often form small groups possessing a commonality which usually opposes other groups.

So it is in medicine. On one side are orthodox practitioners, traditional doctors versed in technology, surgery, and pharmaceuticals. On the other side stand the alternative practitioners: acupuncturists, healing arts specialists, Reiki practitioners, naturopaths, and even some "turncoat" medical doctors. Currently, clear lines have been drawn in the sand. Each side is intransigent, refusing to explore the possible benefits of the opposing camp. To clarify this situation, let me share some personal experiences.

As you are aware, I was born and raised in orthodoxy. My practice includes the most technologically advanced of all cardiac procedures—angioplasties, stents, atherectomies, and radio frequency ablations. When I began to incorporate alternative approaches such as vitamins, minerals, herbs, and supplements into my traditional practice, I was swiftly ostracized by the local medical community. I became practically a pariah, and previously supportive physicians ceased to send me their patients. As a consultant, I am, to a large extent, dependent upon referrals for my medical and financial survival. You might imagine, therefore, that the abrupt termination of a flow of patients was not without pain. I spoke with my peers, attempting to share the vision that I enjoyed. Their minds and hearts were sealed. I found it nearly impossible to convince them that I was not abandoning the "faith" of orthodox medicine, but rather I had found other ways to help heal our mutual patients. During heated discussions these doctors would often refer to the lack of scientific evidence supporting any use of vitamins, minerals, herbs, supplements, or even stress-reduction techniques.

I responded to these claims with two major arguments. First, there is a large body of data supporting the use of natural remedies in the treatment of a whole host of disease states. There are also substantial data showing the preventative benefits of various vitamins such as E and C. Although I presented articles to many of these physicians, the responses were often similar: "The study is too small. This is not a good enough journal. It is just one study!" The excuses for closed-mindedness are seemingly endless.

My other approach in defending my position regards science itself. Science is overrated. Sure, without science we would lack many modern miraculous devices in both medicine and other arenas, but science is not everything. Art and instinct are often vastly greater tools for even orthodox physicians in the management of patients. To understand this, one must simply attend any large medical conference. Typically, the highlight of a medical meeting is an expert panel debate. During these debates, world-renowned leaders in a given field will discuss and debate various treatment strategies with regard to a particular ailment. I have listened with bewilderment as the experts espouse even antithetical approaches to a simple ailment. At times, I have left these debates totally nonplussed—feeling impotent and unsure of how to approach a disorder which I had previously treated with great confidence. After serious reflection, however, I have realized that even in the face of scientific dogma, there is no right or wrong in relation to the treatment of most disease processes. Thus, when physicians rely on science as their foundation of strength and proof that what they do is right, they are wearing blinders, ignoring the real "truth" of medicine. Medicine is an art. Ninety percent of what we do is based upon instinct and gut, rather than scientific dogma.

Alternative practitioners are often no less narrow-minded than the traditionalists. When opponents of traditional medicine make claims that many bypass surgeries are performed unnecessarily—solely for the financial enhancement of heart surgeons, some people argue—they could not be farther from the truth. The reality is that most bypass surgeries, although not performed to save lives, are undertaken as a means of helping patients. These surgeries are carried out because doctors believe in their hearts that their patients are better off with them than without them. There is no malevolence and no greed involved in this decision-making process. There is also no science.

To close the gap between orthodox and alternative medicine, traditionalists must own up to their reliance upon instinct as their most powerful tool in healing. Once they accept this truth, they will be unable to fight alternative approaches on the grounds of absent scientific data.

By the same token, for the alternative medicine practitioners to embrace orthodox doctors, they must acknowledge the veritable miracles of modern medicine. Bypass surgery can, at times, save lives. Surgery can cure cancers. Chemotherapy, at times, can also cure cancers. Alternative medicine practitioners must accept and even embrace the benefits of modern medicine.

Within the past year, I had the privilege of caring for a prominent alternative medicine physician, Dr. Robert Willix, a previously preeminent heart surgeon who left the world of orthodox medicine to pursue a path of purely alternative practice. He became expert in the field of Ayurvedic medicine and opened an office in Boca Raton where he treats and helps many patients. One day I received a telephone call from Dr. Willix's wife. She was terrified. Her husband was experiencing chest discomfort and weakness. His color was ashen and his pulse thready. I instructed her to have him go to Boca Raton Community Hospital's emergency room, as I believed he was experiencing a heart attack. Unfortunately, I was correct. Dr. Willix was having a small inferior wall myocardial infarction (a heart attack on the under surface of his heart). I remember talking with him in the emergency room, saying, "You do believe in *integrative* medicine, don't you?" A simple *no* was his response. As the moments passed, however, he appeared to reflect deeply, and then accepted a more traditional approach to his disease. I placed him on intravenous nitroglycerine, intravenous heparin, and gave him aspirin. His pain abated. Dr. Willix was fortunate. He had had a very small heart attack. He agreed to perform a stress test prior to his discharge which, as he predicted, demonstrated merely a small heart attack. There was no evidence of any other coronary artery disease. He left the hospital and has been pain-free since then.

Dr. Willix exercises vigorously, eats impeccably, and is amazingly fit emotionally, physically, and spiritually. He acknowledges that he had been working extraordinarily long and arduous hours at the time of his heart attack. Since then, he has achieved greater balance in his life. He has also accepted a more balanced perspective with regard to healing. Although he still practices alternative medicine, Dr. Willix appreciates what modern medicine has to offer. If medical practitioners wish to improve the state of healing in America, we must all become more like Dr. Willix. We must put aside our weapons of insecurity and hostility, and learn to appreciate what each group and every individual healer has to offer. Only through this harmonious interaction of healers will Americans reap the rewards of a truly integrated health care system.

On a small level, I have tried to accomplish this task by forming The Baum Center for Integrative Heart Care. I have had the good fortune of bringing together a dedicated group of eclectic healers. At our center, we have a stress-reduction program in which mindfulness-based stress reduction, body scan, meditation, Reiki, and freeze frame are taught. T'ai Chi and yoga classes are offered, along with instruction in aerobic exercise and resistance training. The center also has a full-time dietitian and licensed nutritionist who advises patients on how to achieve optimum nutritional states and weight loss (when necessary). I feel fortunate that everyone who works at the center is a dedicated, highly educated, inspired professional in his or her chosen field. Implementing truly integrative heart health care would not be possible without their input and caring.

My role, of course, includes ensuring the safety of our patients from an orthodox medical perspective. In addition to making recommendations regarding vitamin, mineral, and nutrient supplements, I also guard the health of our patients by utilizing orthodox medical tests and procedures when necessary.

You can see that we view optimal health in multifaceted terms. Attention to merely one or two isolated components leaves individuals incomplete and unprotected from the ravages of disease. I do not mean to imply, however, that if one utilizes each of the aforementioned components of health promotion, he will be rendered immune to disease. I am certain, though, that as we strengthen our emotions, spirits, and physical beings, we become vitalized and increasingly resistant to stress and illness. It is my dream, and the dream of those in our center, that in the not-too-distant future, all doctors will acknowledge the value of interacting with a variety of healers linked by the common goal of health and healing. We will then be capable of achieving optimal health care.

Good health to you all.

Suggested Reading

Balsch, James F., Phyllis A. Balsch, C.N.C.; *Prescription for Nutritional Healing*; Avery Publishing Group; 1993.

Benson, Herbert, M.D.; *The Relaxation Response;* Avon; 1975.

Braverman, Eric R., M.D., Matthew Taub, M.D.; *The Amazing Way to Reverse Heart Disease Naturally;* Keats Publishing Group; 1996.

Chopra, Depak, M.D.; *Ageless Body, Timeless Mind, The Quantum Alternative to Growing Old;* Harmony Books; 1993.

Coleman, Donald A., M.D., Nancy Szeman, R.D., C.D.E.; *The Top 100 International Low-Fat Recipes*; Time-Life Books, Inc.; 1996.

The Complete German Commission E Monographs, Therapeutic Guide to Herbal Medicines; Senior Editor, Mark Blumenthal; American Botanical Council; 1998.

Cranton, Elmore, M.D., Arlene Brecher; *Bypassing Bypass, The New Technique of Chelation Therapy;* Stein & Day; 2d edition; 1984; 1990.

Crayhon, Robert, M.S.; *The Carnitine Miracle;* Evans and Co; 1998.

D'Adamo, Peter J., N.D., Catherine Whitney; *Four Blood Types, Four Diets, Eat Right for Your Type, The Invidualized Diet Solution to Staying Healthy, Living Longer and Achieving Your Ideal Weight;* Putnam; 1996.

Danbrot, Margaret; *The New Cabbage Soup Diet;* Lynn Sanberg, Book Associates; 1997.

Danniston, Denise, Peter McWilliams; *The Transcendental Meditation Book;* Warner Books; 1975.

Eades, Michael R., M.D., Mary Dan Eades, M.D.; *Protein Power;* Bantam Books; 1996.

Fritzweiss, Rudolph, M.D.; *Herbal Medicine;* Beaconsfield Publishers, Ltd.; 1988; 4th edition; 1996.

Goldberg, Burton, Editors of *Alternative Medicine Digest; Alternative Medicine Guide to Heart Disease;* Future Medicine Publishing, Inc.; 1988.

Kabat-Zinn, John, Ph.D.; *Full Catastrophe Living;* Dell; 1990.

Kirschmann, Gayla J., John. D. Kirschmann; *Nutrition Almanac;* McGraw Hill; 1996.

Klein, Alan; *The Healing Power of Humor;* Jeremy P. Tarcher/Putnam; 1989.

Lipetz, Philip, Monika Pichler; *Naturally Slim and Powerful;* Andrews McMeel, a Universal Press Syndicated Co.; 1997.

Mabey, Richard; *The New Age Herbalist;* Simon & Schuster; 1988.

McArdle, William, Frank Katch, Victor Katch; *Exercise Physiology, Energy, Nutrition and Human Performance;* Williams Wilkins; 1996.

McCulley, Kilmer S., M.D.; *The Homocysteine Revolution;* Keats Publishing; 1997.

Mills, Simon Y.; *The Essential Book of Herbal Medicine;* Penguin Publishing; 1991.

Murray, Michael T., N.D.; *Encyclopedia of Nutritional Supplements;* Prima Publishing; 1996.

Murray, Michael T., N.D.; *The Healing Power of Herbs;* Prima Publishing; 1992; 2d edition; 1995.

Murray, Michael T., N.D.; *Heart Disease and High Blood Pressure, How You Can Benefit from Diet, Vitamins, Minerals, Herbs, Exercise and Other Natural Methods;* Prima Publishing; 1997.

Murray, Michael T., N.D.; *Natural Alternatives to Over the Counter and Prescription Drugs;* William Morrow; 1994.

Murray, Michael T., N.D., Joseph Pizzorno, N.D.; *Encyclopedia of Natural Medicine;* Prima Publishing; 1991.

Ornish, Dean, M.D.; *Dr. Dean Ornish's Program for Reversing Heart Disease;* Ballantine Books; 1990.

Ornish, Dean, M.D.; *Love and Survival;* HarperCollins; 1997.

Ortiz, Elizabeth Lambert; *The Encyclopedia of Herbs, Spices and Flavorings;* Dorling Kindersley; 1992.

Peckenpaugh, Nancy J., Charlotte M. Polman; *Nutrition, Essentials and Diet Therapy;* Saunders; 1995.

Pedersen, Mark; *Nutritional Herbology, A Reference Guide to Herbs;* Wittman; 1994.

Pollock, Michael L., Ph.D.; Jack Wilmore, Ph.D.; *Exercise in Health and Disease;* Saunders; 1990.

Price, Shirley, Len Price; *Aromatherapy for Health Professionals;* Churchill Livingstone; 1995.

Rosenfeld, Isadore, M.D.; *Dr. Rosenfeld's Guide to Alternative Medicine;* Random House; 1996.

Rothfeld, Glenn S., M.D., Suzanne Luvert; *Natural Medicine for Heart Disease, The Best Alternative Methods For Prevention and Treatment;* Rodale Press; 1996.

Sachs, Judith; *Natural Medicine for Heart Disease;* Dell; 1996.

Sears, Barry, Ph.D., with Bill Lawrence; *The Zone;* Regan Books; 1995.

Selye, Hans; *Stress Without Distress;* Cygnet Press; 1974.

Shute, Evan V., F.R.S.C.(C); *The Heart and Vitamin E;* Keats Publishing; 1956; most recent edition; 1977.

Tyler, Varoe, Ph.D.; *The Honest Herbal;* Pharmaceutical Products Press; 1982; 3d edition; 1993.

Weil, Andrew, M.D.; *Health and Healing;* Houghton Mifflin; 1983; most recent edition; 1995.

Weil, Andrew, M.D.; *Spontaneous Healing;* Fawcett Columbine; 1995.

Wildwood, Chrissie; *Encyclopedia of Aromatherapy;* Healing Arts Press; 1996.

Glossary

A-A interval: the time between two electrical discharges of the atria.

Adrenergic (or sympathetic) nervous system: the portion of the autonomic nervous system responsible for the stress-activated "fight or flight" reaction.

A-H interval: the time from electrical activity of the low right atrium to electrical contact with the HIS bundle.

Alph-linolenic acid: an omega-3 essential fatty acid.

Amino acids: the building blocks of all proteins.

Angina pectoris: a squeezing, pressure-like sensation or pain in the mid-portion of the chest caused by constricted coronary arteries.

Angiogram (cardiac catheterization): a procedure in which a cardiologist punctures the artery in the groin and passes fine tubes into the arteries of the heart to define their anatomy.

Aortic regurgitation: leaking of the aortic valve.

Aortic stenosis: narrowing of the aortic valve.

Atrial fibrillation: an abnormal, rapid heart rhythm emanating from the upper chambers of the heart.

Atrioventricular node (A-V node): an electrical filter that creates a slight pause during each heartbeat.

Atrioventricular valves: the valves that separate the atria and ventricles, called the "tricuspid valve" and the "mitral valve."

Balloon mitral valvuloplasty: a procedure in which a single or double balloon is passed through the artery in the groin to the mitral valve and then expanded, cracking the valve open to increase the size of the mitral valve orifice.

Bruce protocol (stress test): a test that uses a series of three-minute stages of walking on a treadmill to assess the heart's ability to respond to physical exertion.

Carbohydrates: compounds made up of the sugars and starches.

Cardiac catheterization (angiogram): a procedure in which a cardiologist punctures the artery in the groin and passes fine tubes into the arteries of the heart to define their anatomy.

Chelation therapy: utilizes intravenous EDTA as a means of removing "free" metal ions (excess iron, copper, and calcium) from the body in an attempt to limit their free-radical-damaging effects on our arteries.

Cholesterol: a type of lipid we need to make our cell membranes pliable, our nerve tissue functional, and to synthesize steroid hormones. High levels can lead to coronary artery disease.

Congestive heart failure: a condition in which the heart, working as a pump, is unable to keep up with the demands placed upon it.

Cor bovinum **(cow heart):** a condition in which the left ventricle becomes hugely enlarged, generally a result of aortic regurgitation or leaking.

Coronary artery bypass grafting (CABG, also often known as ACB or aortocoronary bypass): a surgical procedure during which new blood vessels are attached to arteries feeding the heart to circumvent prior blockage and deliver adequate supplies of blood and oxygen to the heart muscle. The patient's own blocked blood vessels are not replaced; they are simply bypassed.

DHA (docosahexaenoic acid): an omega-3 fatty acid possessing many health benefits.

Diastole: when the heart rests between beats.

Dilated cardiomyopathy (DCM): a condition in which the heart becomes enlarged, weakened, and flabby. DCM is an insidious disease often culminating in severe congestive heart failure.

Echocardiogram (ECHO): the ECHO is a "fancy" ultrasound, in which sound waves are sent to different structures, and then bounce back with varying intensities. The pattern of their return to the recording device reveals either the physical structure under study or its blood flow.

EDRF (endothelial-derived relaxing factor): a powerful natural dilator (expander of blood vessels).

Electrocardiogram (ECG or EKG): a test in which a series of ten electrodes are positioned on the chest, arms, and legs to record the heart's electrical forces on paper.

EPA (eicosapentaenoic acid): an omega-3 fatty acid possessing numerous health benefits.

EPS: electrophysiologic studies which examine the electrical functioning of the heart.

Essential amino acids: the nine amino acids we cannot create in our bodies and must obtain from the diet.

Essential fatty acids: alpha-linolenic (omega-3) and linoleic (omega-6), are "essential" fatty acids, meaning our bodies are incapable of producing them and so we must obtain them from our diet.

Factor 7: a clotting factor; an elevated level has been shown to increase the frequency of coronary artery disease.

Fiber: also known as roughage, fiber is an indigestible form of carbohydrates.

Fibrinogen: a blood component that helps promote clotting; elevated levels are an independent risk factor for cardiovascular disease.

Glucose: the form of sugar that is our body's most important fuel.

HDL (high-density lipoproteins): the "good" cholesterol, the lipoprotein that brings fat back to the liver to be metabolized.

Heart attack (myocardial infarction): the result of an active blockage in an artery. The common denominator of all heart attack victims is the presence of a blood clot inside a blood vessel. A heart attack results in death of a portion of the heart muscle.

HIS bundle: the electrical "wire" that connects the atria and ventricles.

Homocysteine: a by-product of amino acid metabolism; an elevated level is a newly appreciated risk factor for coronary artery disease.

H-V interval: the time from onset of electrical activity in the HIS bundle to onset of electrical activity in the ventricles.

Hypertrophic cardiomyopathies (HCM): heart muscle diseases in which the muscle becomes thickened.

Idiopathic dilated cardiomyopathy (IDCM): a common type of DCM in which the heart becomes enlarged, weakened, and flabby from an unknown cause.

Inotropy: the heart's ability to squeeze.

Insufficient valve (or regurgitant): a leaky heart valve.

Ischemia: lack of adequate blood flow or oxygen supply.

LDL (low-density lipoproteins): the "bad" cholesterol, the lipoprotein that carries cholesterol to various parts of the body.

Left atrium: the upper chamber of the heart that receives "clean" or oxygenated blood from the lungs.

Left ventricle: the lower chamber of the heart that receives blood from the left atrium, ejects blood into the aorta, and then onward to the body and brain for sustenance.

Linoleic acid: an omega-6 essential fatty acid.

Lipids: fats.

LPa (lipoprotein a): a particularly sticky form of LDL; an elevated level of LPa is an independent risk factor for coronary artery disease.

Minerals: Inorganic substances required in small quantities to satisfy the needs of our enzymatic machinery.

Mitochondria: our cells' energy-producing organelles.

Mitral regurgitation: leaking of the mitral valve.

Mitral stenosis: a condition in which the mitral valve (which separates the left atrium from the left ventricle) is narrowed.

Mitral valve: the valve that separates the left atrium from the left ventrical.

Mitral valve prolapse (MVP, also known as Barlow syndrome): a disorder of the mitral valve in which the valve leaflets bow back (i.e., prolapse) into the left atrium during ventricular systole (contraction).

Monounsaturated fats: fats containing a single double bond, like oleic acid in canola and olive oil. These are healthful oils.

Myocardial infarction (heart attack): the result of an active blockage in an artery. The common denominator of all heart attack victims is the presence of a blood clot inside a blood vessel. A heart attack results in death of a portion of the heart muscle.

National Cholesterol Education Program (NCEP): a panel associated with the National Institutes of Health.

Omega-3 fatty acid: an unsaturated fat, having its first double bond at the third carbon atom.

Omega-6 fatty acid: an unsaturated fat, having its first double bond at the sixth carbon atom.

Oxidized LDL: damaged LDL cholesterol that adheres to arterial walls and contributes to the buildup of plaque.

P-wave: the electrical impulse that initiates the normal heartbeat.

Parasympathetic nervous system: the portion of the autonomic nervous system that balances the sympathetic nervous system and promotes relaxation.

Pericardium: the thin, smooth, two-layered sac that surrounds the heart.

PET (positron emission tomography) scan: an expensive test that detects reduced blood flow (ischemia) and currently adds little to other, more traditional stress tests.

Plaque: an accumulation of oxidized LDL cholesterol (and other substances) on the inner wall of an artery that clogs the artery and can result in the development of angina or heart attacks.

Plasminogen activator inhibitor 1 (PAI-1): a blood factor; when PAI-1 levels are elevated, a decrease in fibrinolytic activity may ensue, possibly resulting in blood clots.

Polyunsaturated fats: fats containing two or more double bonds, which are very susceptible to oxidation. These are generally more healthful than saturated fats.

Protein: a dietary macromolecule built of amino acids.

PR interval: the pause in a normal heartbeat occuring between atrial and ventricular excitation.

Purkinje fibers: small fibers comprising the minor "wires" delivering electrical impulses to the heart muscle (ventricles).

QRS complex: the EKG part of the heartbeat in which electrical activity of the ventricles produces the major squeeze of the heart.

Regurgitant (or insufficient) valve: a leaky heart valve.

Restenosis: renarrowing of an artery or valve after a corrective procedure (such as angioplasty) has been performed.

Restrictive cardiomyopathy (RCM): an abnormality of the heart muscle in which it is unable to fill with blood appropriately.

Right atrium: the upper chamber of the heart that collects "dirty" or unoxygenated blood from the veins.

Right ventricle: the lower chamber of the heart that receives blood from the right atrium, and sends the blood toward the lungs.

Saturated fats: fats that contain no double bonds; they are usually solid at room temperature and considered to be unhealthful.

SBE (subacute bacterial endocarditis): a potentially serious infection of the heart valves.

Silent ischemia: a condition in which there is no pain (like angina), yet the individual suffers from significant coronary arterial blockage.

Sinoatrial node (the S-A node): the heart's natural pacemaker.

ST segment: the portion of the heartbeat that is the major focus of attention during exercise stress testing.

Stenosis: narrowing of a heart artery or valve.

Stress test: a test that assesses the heart's ability to respond to physical exertion or an injected substance that simulates exercise.

Sympathetic (or adrenergic) nervous system: the part of the autonomic nervous system responsible for the stress-activated "fight or flight" reaction.

Syncope: fainting.

Systole: when the ventricles contract, i.e., beat.

T-wave: the part of the heartbeat during which the heart's electrical charge is changed so that it is ready to accept its next electrical impulse.

TEE (transesophageal echocardiogram): a test in which a Doppler probe is positioned at the tip of a long tube, which needs to be swallowed in order to view the heart from *behind*, with the probe resting within the esophagus (the pipe connecting the mouth to the stomach).

TIAs (transient ischemic attacks): ministrokes.

Trans-fatty acids: fats created by hydrogenation that take on characteristics even worse than those of the saturated fatty acids, increasing total cholesterol and LDL and lowering the heart-protective HDL cholesterol.

Tricuspid stenosis (TS): narrowing of the tricuspid valve, usually resulting from rheumatic heart disease.

Tricuspid regurgitation (TR): leaking of the tricuspid valve.

Tricuspid valve: the valve that separates the right atrium from the right ventrical.

Type A personality: this personality is typically angry, pressured, visibly tense, and intolerant; possessing type A personality is a risk factor for coronary artery disease.

Ultrafast CT: a test utilizing an electron beam that searches for abnormal calcium deposits within the coronary arteries.

Unstable angina: A pattern of angina which is rapidly progressive, resulting from a decrease in supply of blood to the heart, leaving it starved for oxygen. The arteries of an unstable angina patient have experienced an abrupt event, such as the rupture of a previously solid plaque, often with the formation of a clot on top of a prior plaque.

Vasoconstriction: tightening of blood vessels.

VEG-F (vascular endothelial growth factor): an experimental gene therapy protein that is injected directly into the heart to stimulate the growth of new coronary arteries.

Ventricles: the lower chambers of the heart.

Ventricular systole: when the ventricles contract, i.e., beat.

Vitamins: substances we cannot create in our bodies and thus must be consumed. They enable our enzymatic systems to function appropriately.

Abnormal Heart Rhythms and Their Treatments

This appendix addresses diverse electrophysiologic ailments, which will be broken into: (1) the bradycardias, or slow heart rhythms, and (2) tachycardias, or fast heart rhythms. Along with these ailments, various therapeutic treatment options will be discussed. This appendix can be used as a reference guide for patients with electrical abnormalities of the heart.

Bradycardias

You may recall from Chapter 2 ("The Heart in Harmony") that the heart has its own natural intrinsic pacemaker. This is called the sinus node. Normally, the sinus node fires 60 to 100 times a minute, producing a heart rate of 60 to 100 beats per minute. This is the normal range of heart rates. At times, however, things can go amiss and the heart rate can be significantly lower than 60 beats per minute. When this occurs, a "bradycardia" is produced.

There are two basic mechanisms that cause bradycardias. The first is an abnormality of impulse formation, which really means that the sinus node is not doing its job. It fails to fire at an appropriate rate.

The second is a failure of atrial-ventricular conduction. This means that although the sinus node is doing its job, the electrical circuitry of the heart is having a problem. The heart's electrical problem is not allowing the sinus node's impulse to traverse the electrical wiring in order to cause a firing (and resultant beating) of the ventricles.

Whether the first or second cause exists is irrelevant, relative to the symptoms that can occur. Symptoms caused by a slow heart rate include lightheadedness, chest pain, or a failure of the heart muscle to function effectively, which can lead to congestive heart failure or simply fatigue. All of these are caused by too little blood reaching the organ in question, i.e., the brain or the heart. Obviously, there is a whole series of reasons why people can become lightheaded or have chest pain or even have heart failure and it is therefore incumbent upon the physician to ferret out the data available to him in order to conclude that the symptoms are, in fact, caused by bradycardia.

What are the typical causes of these bradycardias? Aside from intrinsic heart disease, there are other phenomena that can lead to bradycardias. These include certain prescription medications, an underactive thyroid (hypothyroidism), a low temperature (hypothermia), an elevated potassium, and autonomic imbalance, meaning that the sympathetic and parasympathetic nervous systems are not appropriately regulated. The parasympathetic nervous system slows the heart rate. When it is overactive, a bradycardia can result, and symptoms from that bradycardia then ensue.

When a patient comes to the emergency room with any of the above-mentioned symptoms caused by a bradycardia, the first and most logical step we take is to increase his heart rate. We can accomplish this with either a temporary pacemaker or the administration of IV medications such as Atropine and Isoproterenol. If the patient's problem is permanent, meaning that there is no reversible cause identified, then he will undergo a permanent pacemaker implantation. (This procedure will be described later in this section.)

Many different types of pacemakers are currently available. The one that would be most often implanted in a patient with an intact sinus node (meaning that he is capable of generating sinus rhythm) would be a dual-chamber pacemaker, one that senses and paces both the upper and the lower chambers of the heart in synchrony.

Now for those extraordinarily courageous readers among you, we will examine several different causes of bradycardias and their respective treatments.

1. Failure of Impulse Formation, or a failure of the sinus node to function appropriately. When the sinus rate falls below 60 beats per minute, a sinus bradycardia results. This is often a benign finding. It occurs extremely frequently in trained athletes, and they are usually asymptomatic. That is, they are totally unaware of their slow heart rate, and do not have any of the symptoms mentioned previously. This form of sinus bradycardia results from increased vagal tone (increased parasympathetic tone).

Sinus bradycardia also occurs very commonly during sleep. In fact, most people have heart rates that drop to the forties and even thirties at some point during their sleep cycle. This is absolutely inconsequential and nothing to worry about.

There are other times, however, when the failure of impulse formation can cause serious consequences, as in certain types of heart attacks (like an inferior wall myocardial infarction). In this situation, there is an increased vagal tone from the heart attack itself. When this occurs, a patient's heart rate can become dangerously slow. The patients may require drug therapy or even a temporary pacemaker. Fortunately, this form of bradycardia is often reversible. As the person recovers from his heart attack, his heart rate will generally return to normal.

Management of sinus bradycardias depends upon the presence or absence of symptoms. When symptoms are present, reversible factors, if any, should be eliminated. If there is nothing obvious that can be reversed and symptoms persist, this patient may require a permanent pacemaker. These are small, computer-like devices which represent man's best attempt to create a mechanical sinus node. They are employed in patients suffering from electrical abnormalities which can lead to fainting, or even death. In the asymptomatic patient, no therapy is warranted.

2. Heart Block. Heart block occurs when there is a failure of A-V (atrial-ventricular) conduction. This results when the sinus node is functioning appropriately, but the electrical wiring, at some location, has a blocked area that prevents the impulse from traveling where it should. Just as with sinus bradycardias, this can occur during normal and abnormal physiologic states. In a normal circumstance, there is an increase in vagal (or parasympathetic) tone. Once again, this can occur in a well-trained athlete or during periods of sleep. When there is an abnormal pathologic state, and no reversible factor is noted, patients may require permanent pacing for this problem.

Whether or not a patient receives a pacemaker depends upon several factors, including his symptoms, the type of block, and the clinical setting of the block: There are three major types of A-V block: first degree, second degree, and third degree. These terms are used very commonly in medical practice and can be very frightening to patients, so here's what they mean:

    a. **First degree A-V block.** This form of block is completely benign, never produces symptoms, and never requires therapy. It refers to a prolonged PR interval.
    b. **Second degree A-V block.**
      1) **Type 1.** This is usually benign and usually asymptomatic. It is extremely rare to require any therapeutic intervention. Known as Wenckebach block, it refers to a progressively longer PR interval which leads to periodic "dropped" beats
      2) **Type 2.** This is much less common than Type 1 second degree A-V block. It is also more malignant. It implies a block at a lower level along the conduction system. Usually, these patients have underlying heart disease and they require permanent pacemakers. Permanent pacemakers will protect them against future fainting spells.
    c. **Third degree A-V block.** This is also known as complete heart block. These patients usually require permanent pacemakers unless there is a reversible cause such as Lyme disease or an acute heart attack.

Bundle Branch Block

    d. **Complete bundle branch block.** Although this condition does not represent a true rhythm disturbance, it occurs frequently and can create fear in patients or family members.
      1) **Right bundle branch block** occurs when the right branch of our heart's electrical wire does not function as well as the left. Usually, this condition is devoid of any adverse consequences. Although its name may be frightening, it is generally a totally harmless condition.
      2) **Left bundle branch block.** This obviously results from an inadequacy in the left bundle branch. This condi-

tion is often associated with some form of underlying heart problem. Having this block, however, does *not* automatically imply that a pacemaker is in your future. Usually, people with this disorder are evaluated with stress tests and echocardiograms. If these tests are normal, no further action needs to be taken.

Permanent Pacemakers

At this point, it is important to explain a little about permanent pacemakers. Permanent pacemakers are implanted in approximately 300,000 people per year in America. There are two major types of permanent pacemakers, single chamber and dual chamber. Single chamber devices pace only the ventricles; that is, they stimulate the lower chambers of the heart. Dual chamber pacemakers stimulate both the upper and the lower chambers of the heart—the upper chambers are stimulated first, then a pause, and then they stimulate the lower chambers. Dual chamber pacemakers truly try to reproduce the normal physiology of the heart's electrical circuitry.

When patients do not have the ability to have their atria paced—for instance, when they are in atrial fibrillation—they require single chamber pacemakers. When they can be paced, they usually require dual chamber pacemakers. The implantation procedure is fairly simple, at least from the perspective of the surgeon. Obviously, from the patient's perspective, it is an operation and, therefore, carries with it emotional and physical consequences that can be very meaningful. From a surgical standpoint, however, the pacemaker implantation entails the following: The patient is brought to an operating suite, lightly sedated. General anesthesia is not necessary. The upper chest region is prepared and draped in a sterile fashion. Subsequently, the surgeon enters the vein under the clavicle (collarbone) and passes wires to the heart. They are positioned to maintain stability and appropriate electrical firing. The surgeon then forms a small pocket (hole) under the skin where he places the pacemaker device (its "brain" and battery).

Previously, pacemakers were huge, unsightly devices. Nowadays, they are extremely small, and therefore, only a minor bulge exists after the pacemaker is inserted in this pocket. A small scar (about 3 inches long) will result from the operation. Patients can usually be sent home on the day following surgery, and they are advised to limit use of their arm, so as not to dislodge the pacemaker wires. Arm limitation is usually advised for only about a week, although at times it can extend up to one month. Careful follow-up of pacemaker function is essential. Pacemakers should be evaluated every one to three months, depending upon how recently they have been implanted. These follow-ups can usually be performed over the telephone. Sometimes, however, patients require on-site evaluations to make certain adjustments in their pacemaker function. No pain or invasion of the body is necessary in pacemaker evaluation, because computers can actually communicate with the pacemaker through the skin. Changes in pacemaker function can even be effected through this communication link.

Complications from pacemaker insertions are uncommon, but can include infections and, rarely, transient lung collapse. Later complications can include rapid heart rhythms which are actually provoked by pacemakers, but these can be prevented by adjusting the pacemaker parameters. Additionally, "pacemaker syndrome" can occur in patients with single chamber pacemakers. This is manifested by lightheadedness, shortness of breath, and fatigue. Dual chamber pacemaker patients do not run the risk of developing this problem.

Palpitations, APCs, and PVCs

Palpitations occur when a patient has an abnormal sensation in either his chest or his throat. This abnormal sensation is usually described as a fluttering feeling. Palpitations is a general term describing a general symptom. When we evaluate patients with this symptom, we are often unable to discover any cause. There are times, however, that patients have underlying electrical occurrences which lead to the palpitations. The most benign of these occurrences are the APCs and PVCs. APCs, or atrial premature contractions, are "extra beats" emanating from the upper chambers of the heart. They are extremely common. One study showed that they occur in only 0.4 percent of asymptomatic healthy men in the Air Force; however, this was a limited EKG analysis. In other studies, APCs have been found to be much more common; some studies approaching 50 to 60 percent of normal patients.

There are numerous precipitators of APCs—alcohol, tobacco, caffeine, fever, emotional stress, and fatigue. These things should be avoided, when possible, in patients with symptoms of APCs. The therapy for APCs is rooted in reassurance—often the most important medicine a doctor can give his patient. Patients are often extremely frightened by the unusual sensation of APCs, and feel it must imply that their hearts are about to stop. If a good dose of reassurance can be administered, patients often will be able to ignore these occasional palpitations and lead a perfectly normal life. At times, beta blocker drugs are used when reassurance is inadequate.

We have noted, in the world of natural medicine, that magnesium supplementation can also be of great benefit to many patients with palpitations resulting from APCs.

PVCs, or premature ventricular contractions, are "extra beats" that emanate from the bottom chambers (the ventricles). These, too, are extremely common, although perhaps less common than APCs. In the absence of underlying heart disease, no increased risk of dying or having an adverse cardiac event exists in patients who have PVCs. It is interesting to note that PVCs increase as we get older. They also occur more frequently in pregnant women and in premenopausal women.

Even when PVCs are strung together in what are called "salvos" of three to five beats, in the absence of underlying structural heart disease, there is no increased risk to the patient. When patients have chronic cardiac disease, the increase in frequency of PVCs, or the salvos of PVCs, increases the risk of mortality. Treating these PVCs, however, does *not* necessarily lower the mortality.

This represents one of the dilemmas facing modern cardiologists. In fact, in a landmark study (CAST, or Cardiac Arrhythmia Suppression Trial), patients with prior heart attacks and asymptomatic PVCs were given specific medicines to suppress these PVCs. The trial was prematurely aborted, as it was found that the patients given these drugs had a higher risk of dying than the patients who were not given the medicines. This trial exemplifies the benefits of "science" in medicine. Doctors' perceptions that these medications would save lives were proved to be wrong. CAST saved countless lives by teaching doctors to avoid powerful anti-arrythmic pharmaceuticals in this group of patients.

Tachycardias

Tachycardias, rapid heart rhythms, can emanate from either the upper or the lower chambers of the heart. They result when the heart rate exceeds 100 beats per minute. The upper chamber rhythm disturbances are called the "supraventricular tachycardias," because they come from above the ventricle. There are numerous types of supraventricular tachycardias. The more common ones will now be described:

1. **Sinus Tachycardia.** The sinus node can sometimes fire too frequently. When this occurs, a tachycardia ensues, and this is called sinus tachycardia. Generally, it is caused by an underlying condition such as a fever or anemia or hyperthyroidism—when the thyroid is functioning too actively. In situations where there is a sinus tachycardia, the general rule of thumb is to treat the underlying cause. For instance, if the thyroid is too active, make it less active. If there is a fever, lower the fever; and if there is an anemia, treat the cause of the anemia and, when absolutely necessary, give a transfusion. Sinus tachycardia is, in and of itself, benign. The underlying cause is the problem.

2. **A-V Nodal Reentry Tachycardia (AVNRT).** This is the most common cause of paroxysmal supraventricular tachycardia (PSVT). Paroxysmal supraventricular tachycardias do just what their name states: they occur in paroxysms or brief bursts. They have an abrupt onset and offset and they are supraventricular; that is, they occur above the ventricles. AVNRT is the most common cause of paroxysmal supraventricular tachycardia, occurring in 60 percent of all cases. This type of tachycardia can be visualized as a circuit with two pathways. There is one that goes forward (or anterograde), and this has properties where the impulse travels very slowly but recovers very quickly, enabling a new impulse to travel down this pathway. The backward or "retrograde" pathway has opposite characteristics. In this pathway, the impulse can travel very rapidly, but it takes a long time for the pathway to recover excitability in order to allow another impulse to enter it. The usual precipitator of this heart rhythm disturbance, AVNRT, is an APC. What happens when an APC occurs is

that these two pathways or "dual pathways" are in different physio-logic states. The one that travels backward, or retrograde, cannot accept a beat because it has a long period of time before it can accept a new impulse. The forward, or anterograde pathway, having a short recovery time, accepts this beat and the impulse travels slowly down this path. It then meets the retrograde pathway and travels backward up this path. A circuit ensues, and a rapid rhythm will take place. Usually, the rate is around 130–190 beats per minute. The EKG is fairly diagnostic (P-waves are not observed).

Usually, the only symptom from this tachycardia is palpitations. Occasionally, people become mildly lightheaded. It is extremely rare for someone to faint as a consequence of this rhythm disturbance. Various precipitators of the rhythm disturbance include smoking, drinking alcohol, fatigue and stress. Patients who are prone to AVNRT should avoid these potential precipitators.

As this rhythm disturbance is benign, treatment begins with the most conservative approach: rest is advised. We can then employ "vagotonic" maneuvers. These are techniques designed to increase the parasympathetic (vagal tone). They include massaging one's carotid artery, performing a Valsalva maneuver (where a person bears down by squeezing his abdominal muscles), and coughing. When children experience this rhythm disturbance, they often are treated by immersing their faces in ice-cold water. This action produces a vagal response and can often break the tachycardia. If these maneuvers fail, patients can still, at times, be effectively treated while remaining at home. A single dose of a relaxing medicine and a heart-slowing medicine can be taken. This will usually do the trick.

If these approaches fail, the patient must go to the emergency room to be treated with intravenous medicines like Adenosine, Vera-pamil, or beta blockers. These medications work 90 percent of the time. Extremely rarely, all of these techniques fail. Patients then require a low energy shock to get them out of their tachycardia. When they require a shock, they are first sedated, so they feel no pain whatsoever. In fact, they usually have no memory of the shock. In those patients who absolutely want to or need to avoid the shock, we can sometimes place a temporary pacemaker into their heart and pace the heart at a rapid rate, thus breaking the tachycardia. This is actually a very safe procedure.

The long-term therapy for patients with AVNRT is: (1) avoid precipitators such as smoking, alcohol, and stress, (2) learn to utilize the physiologic maneuvers that we have just described. If this fails, the patient can be given a "cocktail" to include medications such as beta blockers and anxiolytic medications like Valium. These should be used only when the patient has the tachycardia. Rarely do patients have such frequent episodes of these tachycardias that they require chronic drug therapy including medicines like Digoxin, beta blockers, and calcium channel blockers.

Some patients cannot tolerate chronic long-term drug therapy. Other patients want to avoid it. These patients are often excellent candidates for radio frequency ablation (RF ablation). This is a procedure that was already described with our patient Ramon Rodriguez. During RF ablation, a catheter is placed within the heart, and a small area of the "extra" pathway or circuit is burned to eliminate the tachycardia. It is extremely low risk, and there is only about a 1–2 percent chance that the patient may require a permanent pacemaker after this procedure. This is truly a curative procedure and, as such, is immensely satisfying for both the physician and the patient.

3. Wolff-Parkinson-White Syndrome. In this condition, an extra pathway called an "accessory pathway" connects the atria to the ventricles, bypassing the A-V node. The accessory pathway is also called a "bypass tract." Bypass tracts represent approximately 25 percent of all paroxysmal supraventricular tachycardias (PSVTs). There are two ways the tracts can conduct: (1) anterograde, or forward from the atria to the ventricles, and, (2) retrograde, or backward from the ventricles to the atria. The most common manner that the pathways conduct is retrograde, i.e., backward from the ventricles to the atria.

When a tachycardia utilizes a retrograde pathway, it is called "orthodromic reentry tachycardia," or ORT. This can often be distinguished from AVNRT by its rapid rate. Orthodromic tachycardias can often exceed 200 beats per minute. The P-waves can also be discernible, occurring after the QRS complexes on the EKG. Usually this type of tachycardia is benign and treated very much like A-V nodal reentry tachycardia, as described above.

The second type of tachycardia is called "antidromic tachycardia," where the impulse is going forward, down the accessory pathway or bypass tract. This results in a "wide complex" tachycardia which possesses a much more ominous appearance on the EKG. It also raises the possibility of more potentially lethal rhythm disturbances that can occur in these patients. Fortunately, it is much rarer than orthodromic tachycardia. Usually, these tachycardias are treated with RF ablation, where the accessory pathway is burned and destroyed. Again, in over 90 percent of patients, this single procedure is curative, and leaves the patients without need for drug therapy and without the fear of fainting or even dying.

4. Other PSVTs. There are a series of other supraventricular tachycardias that represent only 10–15 percent of all PVSTs. They include sinus node reentry, intra-atrial reentry, and automatic ectopic atrial tachycardias. If it is necessary to distinguish among these types of tachycardias for therapeutic reasons, electrophysiologic studies can be definitive. Occasionally, these patients can require radio frequency ablation or chronic drug therapy to manage their troubling symptoms.

5. Nonparoxysmal Supraventricular Tachycardias. These tachycardias occur in a nonparoxysmal fashion—they do not have an abrupt onset or offset, but can have gradual onsets and offsets and can be more chronic. There are three major categories that will be discussed.

    a. **MAT** or "Multifocal Atrial Tachycardia." In this situation, patients with lung disease, specific metabolic disturbances, or electrolyte abnormalities can develop a tachycardia in which there are multiple different types of P-waves, the impulses that are formed from atrial electrical activity. This is a fairly unusual form of tachycardia, and once again therapy is aimed at treating the underlying cause. Occasionally, calcium channel blocker drug therapy can be effective.

    b. **Atrial Flutter.** Atrial flutter is a rapid, regular reentry tachycardia which, of course, emanates from the atria. The atria beat at about 300 times per minute in this tachycardia. Fortunately, the ventricles beat at a much slower rate because they are protected by the A-V node—the heart's natural filter mechanism. Atrial flutter is much less common than paroxysmal supraventricular tachycardias, or even atrial fibrillation, which will be discussed in the next section. It is an extremely rare rhythm in normal patients and usually occurs in patients who have some form of underlying heart disease. Atrial flutter can occur at any age. Common conditions leading to this rhythm disturbance include atrial abnormalities from mitral valve disease, congenital heart disease, and various cardiomyopathies. It is especially common in children who have undergone surgical procedures for complex congenital abnormalities.

We generally treat this rhythm disturbance with medications, and occasionally we utilize a low energy shock to break the rhythm disturbance. As in the case of the paroxysmal supraventricular tachycardias, this rhythm can also be terminated by temporarily pacing the heart at a rapid rate. The good news about this tachycardia is that patients who have it are not at increased risk for clotting and, therefore, do not require long-term anticoagulation therapy.

  c. **Atrial Fibrillation.** Atrial fibrillation is a chaotic rhythm disturbance afflicting some 2 million Americans. It emanates from the upper chambers of the heart. In this rhythm disturbance, the atria are quivering at a rate of 400 to 500 beats per minute. By quivering at this rapid rate, they have no effective squeezing capability and, thus, blood becomes stagnant and easily susceptible to clotting. Atrial fibrillation is age-related, in that it occurs very infrequently in young adults and much more frequently in patients as they reach the age of 70 or greater. In fact, some studies have shown that it occurs in about 10 percent of the population over the age of 70.
  Atrial fibrillation is assessed by cardiologists in the context of its risk. This means that people are broken down into two categories: (1) high risk for clotting and stroke, and (2) low risk for clotting and stroke. This is truly the most important consideration with regard to atrial fibrillation, for it is otherwise not a dangerous rhythm abnormality. It may cause symptoms like shortness of breath, chest discomfort, and fatigue. It is not, however, in and of itself, life-threatening. The major potential complication from atrial fibrillation, however, is that of stroke, where a clot is fired from the atria into the brain. Patients at highest risk for strokes are those with rheumatic heart disease, having a seventeen-fold increase in risk. Patients with idiopathic dilated cardiomyopathies in which the heart muscle is very weak from an unclear cause are also at high risk for stroke.

Other factors known to increase the risk of stroke include an enlarged left atrium, the recent onset of atrial fibrillation, hyperthyroidism, and a prior embolic event (i.e., blood clot).

Patients with atrial fibrillation are evaluated by their cardiologist to determine whether they have any underlying structural heart disease. Echocardiograms and stress tests will usually suffice to determine the general health of a patient's heart. Thyroid function tests (blood tests) are always assessed in patients with atrial fibrillation. An overactive thyroid is one of the reversible causes of this heart rhythm disturbance (as we all recall from one of our prior presidents, George Bush).

When there is no evidence of underlying structural heart disease and the patient has atrial fibrillation, we call this "lone atrial fibrillation." It is more common in young adults. Fortunately, these patients are at very low risk for stroke. Certain precipitators such as cigarettes, alcohol, coffee, stress, and exercise can lead to bouts of atrial fibrillation, especially in the lone atrial fibrillation population. When we uncover underlying precipitators, we advise our patients to avoid them. In patients with lone paroxysmal atrial fibrillation, where episodes of atrial fibrillation come and go, conservative therapy is usually warranted. We recommend lifestyle changes (where appropriate), reassurance, rest, and occasionally anxiolytic medications— medicines such as Valium. We also recommend aspirin. Generally speaking, we do not advise these patients to endure long-term pharmaceutical agents.

In patients who have persistent or chronic atrial fibrillation, the primary goal of the cardiologist is to avoid any complications. Young patients with lone atrial fibrillation have a low risk of stroke and, therefore, require simply an aspirin a day. In those patients with a high risk for stroke, Coumadin should be administered. Coumadin is an oral anticoagulant which is extremely effective at lowering the risk of stroke in atrial fibrillation patients. Numerous studies have documented this, including the SPAF study and the AFASAK study. Patients on anticoagulants have only a 1 or 2 percent risk of stroke, whereas in the absence of anticoagulation, they have a 6 or 7 percent annual risk of stroke. Bleeding complications occur in about 1 or 2 percent of patients on long-term anticoagulation therapy. Of course, it is extremely important to follow the bleeding parameters very closely, and this often requires a blood test every three to six weeks. It is also equally important to have a stable diet—not to be changing the intake of vegetables or alcoholic consumption (unless one has been overimbibing) when a patient is taking Coumadin therapy.

Once we have addressed the potential risks of atrial fibrillation, it then becomes important to address the symptoms of atrial fibrillation. As stated before, patients with atrial fibrillation can develop chest discomfort, shortness of breath, fatigue, and a decreased ability to perform certain exercises they had previously been accustomed to performing. Usually, these symptoms are caused by a rapid heart rate from the atrial fibrillation, and this can be treated with medications which slow the ventricular rate of the patient. These medicines include beta blockers, calcium channel blockers, and Digoxin. When patients cannot tolerate these medications, or when they are ineffective at adequately diminishing the heart rate, radio frequency ablation, once again, can be used to help the patient.

Currently, there are two major types of RF ablation for atrial fibrillation. In the first type, we try gently to burn an area of the heart and, thus, slow the rate of the atrial fibrillation. In the second type, we totally eliminate conduction between the upper and lower chambers of the heart and then implant a permanent pacemaker. In the latter, the patient does become pacemaker-dependent. Although this procedure sounds extreme, it is actually very effective at decreasing the symptoms that can occur with atrial fibrillation. In the future, it is hopeful that we will be able to perform the Maze procedure, where little strips are burned in the atria, eliminating the possibility that atrial fibrillation can ever develop. When this procedure is perfected, it will certainly be a boon to the 2 million Americans that are affected annually from this disorder.

Ventricular Tachycardia and Ventricular Fibrillation

There are about 800,000 heart attack survivors annually in the United States of America. Approximately 10 percent of these, or

80,000, are at increased risk of dying suddenly from a heart rhythm disturbance.

Through the years, cardiologists have wondered how to approach these patients. Should they be treated empirically with drugs in order to limit their risk? In the late 1980s a study called CAST was designed to address this problem. CAST, or Cardiac Arrhythmia Suppression Trial, enrolled patients who had had heart attacks and then developed asymptomatic PVCs, a known predictor of increased risk of dying from cardiac arrhythmias. The patients were placed into two groups: (1) placebo, and (2) drug treatment with anti-arrhythmic medications. To most physicians' surprise, patients in the drug treatment group died prematurely. Consequently, the trial was stopped prematurely. This trial dramatically changed physicians' approaches to heart rhythm disturbances. It became painfully clear that we need to know not only which patients are at increased risk of dying from a rhythm disturbance, but also that the therapy we utilize is effective at preventing the rhythm disturbance and will not kill our patients.

Before we discuss therapy for ventricular tachycardia or ventricular fibrillation, we must first define these terms. Ventricular tachycardia is a rapid rhythm, over 100 beats per minute, which originates in the bottom chambers of the heart. It is an organized rhythm, and is usually a re-entry tachycardia caused by an abnormal circuit in the heart. There are different types of ventricular tachycardia. The most common form is sustained monomorphic ventricular tachycardia, meaning that it is a prolonged episode and it is of uniform quality. This potentially lethal rhythm disturbance is almost always the result of a prior myocardial infarction. Patients with this form of rhythm disturbance should undergo electrophysiologic studies to evaluate appropriate therapeutic interventions. More and more, it is becoming apparent that ICDs (implantable cardioverter defibrillators) will be the mainstay of therapy. These devices are like brilliant pacemakers. They constantly survey the heart's rhythm and deliver shocks to abort any potentially life-threatening rhythm problems. Previous attempts at radio frequency ablation for this type of rhythm disturbance have demonstrated limited value. Drugs for ventricular tachycardia have very common and dangerous side effects and are often incompletely effective. Once again, implantable cardioverted defibrillators are becoming the treatment of choice for this rhythm disturbance.

One form of ventricular tachycardia that bears special mention is *torsade de pointes* (TDP), which means "turning on the point." This is a form of ventricular tachycardia often caused by drugs that we doctors prescribe. The most common medicines that cause this rhythm disturbance are a specific class of anti-arrhythmic agents. TDP can also occur in the setting of low potassium, severely slow heart rhythms, low magnesium, congenital abnormalities and liquid protein diets. This rhythm disturbance must be dealt with immediately or it can become fatal. Remember, removing the underlying cause and administering IV magnesium are the treatments of choice.

Not all ventricular tachycardias are deadly. Special mention should be made of two forms that occur in "normal" hearts. One is a "catecholamine sensitive" ventricular tachycardia, and the other is a "adenosine sensitive" ventricular tachycardia. The first is treated with beta blockers, and the second with calcium channel blockers. Radio frequency ablation has been used to treat both of these rhythm disturbances very effectively.

Ventricular fibrillation is a terminal rhythm disturbance which is chaotic and irregular. Just like atrial fibrillation, where the atria are quivering in an unsynchronized fashion, so too in ventricular fibrillation is the entire heart quivering in an unsynchronized fashion. This rhythm disturbance nearly always leads to sudden cardiac death, and if the patient is not resuscitated very rapidly, death ensues. The usual cause of ventricular fibrillation is an acute ischemic event, where there is a blockage in one of the arteries that feeds the heart. It is the ultimate cause of 25–50 percent of all deaths from cardiomyopathies. In the outpatient setting, ventricular tachycardia is usually the precursor to ventricular fibrillation in cardiac arrest patients. Ventricular tachycardia, if allowed to continue for too long a period of time, can eventually degenerate into ventricular fibrillation and become the patient's fatal rhythm. In ventricular fibrillation, electrophysiologic-guided therapy is more difficult. People with ventricular fibrillation, in the absence of an acute heart attack, generally require an implantable cardioverted defibrillator.

A final condition that can lead to fatal rhythm disturbances is the congenital long QT syndromes. Fortunately, these are rare conditions, as they represent diseases which can kill our most treasured people—our children. Congenital long QT syndromes brutally depict the mind-body relationship. It is in these patients that emotions can directly lead to death. In fact, the saying "scared to death" may have been born of this disorder. The classic description of a child being scolded by his teacher and then falling to the floor dead—literally, dropping dead—represents a description of the long QT syndrome. When children faint, this condition should always be considered. When diagnosed, these children are treated with beta blockers or implantable cardioverter defibrillators. Obviously, psychological counseling is warranted in patients with this disorder and their families.

Generic and Trade Name Drugs

Generic	Pharmaceutical Trade Name
Blood Pressure Pills	
Beta Blockers	
Atenolol	Tenormin
Labetalol	Normodyne Trandate
Metoprolol	Lopressor
Nadolol	Corgard
Oxprenolol	Trasicor
Pindolol	Visken
Propranolol	Inderal, Inderal LA
Timolol	Bolcadren, Betim
Diuretics	
Thiazides	Diuril, Saluric
Chlorothiazide	Hydrodiuril, Esidrix
Hydrochlorothiazide	Oretic, Direma
Bendrofluazide	Aprinox, Berkozide
	Centyl, Neo-Naclex
Chlorthalidone	Hygroton
Indapamide	Lozol, Natrilix
Metolazone	Zaroxolyn, Metenix
Strong Diuretics	
Furosemide, frusemide	Lasix, Dryptal
Bumetanide	Burinex, Bumex
Ethacrynic acid	Edecrin
Diuretics that retain potassium	
Amiloride	Midamor
Spironolactone	Aldactone
Triamterene	Dyrenium Dytac

Generic	Pharmaceutical Trade Name
Thiazide combined with potassium-retaining diuretic	
Nongeneric names	Aldactazide
	Dyazide
	Moduretic, Moduret
Vasodilators (dilate arteries) (pages 000–000)	
Captopril	Capoten
Enalapril	Vasotec
Hydralazine	Apresoline
Nifedipine	Adalat, Procardia
Prazosin	Minipress, Hypovase
Other Antihypertensives	
Clonidine	Catapres
Guanabenz	Wytensin
Methyldopa	Aldomet, Dopamet,
	Hydromet, Medomet
Reserpine	Abicol, Decasepyl,
	Endruronyl, Harmonyl,
	Raudixin, Rautrax,
	Serpasil, others
Drugs Used for Angina	
Beta Blockers See above.	
Calcium Antagonists	
Diltiazem	Cardizem, Tiazac
Nifedipine	Adalat, Procardia
Verapamil	Calan, Isoptin,
	Vasolan
Nitrates	
Nitroglycerine (sublingual)	Nitrostat, Nitro-Bid,
	Others
Isosorbid dinitrate	Coronex, Isordil,
	Sorbitrate, others
	Minitran

Generic	Pharmaceutical Trade Name

Drugs for Heart Failure

Digoxin	Lanoxin, others
Forosemide and other diuretics	See above.
Vasodilators such as Captopril and Enalapril	

Drugs for Abnormal Heart Rhythms (Arrhythmias)

Amiodarone	Cordarone, Cordarone X
Beta-blockers. See above.	
Digoxin	Lanoxin
Disopyramide	Norpace, Rythmodan
Mexiletine	Mexitil
Pronestyl	ProcainSR
Sotalol	Betapace
Tocainide	Tonocard
Quinidine	Cardioquin, Quinidex, Quinate, Biquin Durules others

Drugs That Affect Blood Clotting

Blood thinners: Anticoagulants

Abciximab	Reopro
Aspirin	Aspirin
Clopidogrel	Plavix
Heparin	Heparin
Warfarin	Coumadin, Warfilone, Marevan, others

Drugs That Reduce Cholesterol or Triglycerides

Atorvastatin	Lipitor
Cholestyramine	Questran, Cuemid, Quantalan
Colestipol	Colestid
Gemfibrozil	Lopid
Lovastatin	Mevacor
Pravastatin	Pravachol
Simvastatin	Zocar

Normal Values or Normal Range
of Some Blood Constituents

dl = deciliter = 100 ml of blood
mEq/L = milliequivalent per liter of blood
mmol/L = micromole per liter of blood

	United States		Canada (metric)
Total cholesterol	150 to 200 mg/dL	÷ 38.7 =	3.7 to 5.7 mmol/L
HDL cholesterol	40 to 80 mg/dL	÷ 38.7 =	to 2 mmol/L
Creatinine	Less than 1.4 mg/dL		Less than 130µmol/l
(Test of kidney function)			
Potassium	3.6 to 5.6 mEq/L		4 to 5 mmol/L
Triglycerides	50 to 200 mg/dL	÷ 100 =	0.5 to 2.5 mmol/L

Bibliography

Allan, Robert, Ph.D., Steven Scheidt, M.D.; *Heart and Mind, The Practice of Cardiac Psychology;* Allan and Scheidt; American Psychological Association; 1996.

Balsch, James F., Phyllis A. Balsch, C.N.C.; *Prescription for Nutritional Healing;* Avery Publishing Group; 1993.

Benson, Herbert, M.D.; *The Relaxation Response;* Avon, 1975.

Braunwald, Eugene; *Heart Disease, A Textbook of Cardiovascular Medicine;* Saunders; 1996.

Braverman, Eric R., M.D., Matthew Taub, M.D.; *The Amazing Way to Reverse Heart Disease Naturally, Hypertension and Nutrition;* Keats Publishing; 1996.

Budnick, Herbert N., Ph.D., Scott Robert Hays; *Heart to Heart, A Guide to the Psychological Aspects of Heart Disease;* Health Press; 1997.

Chopra, Deepak, M.D.; *Ageless Body, Timeless Mind, The Quantum Alternative to Growing Old;* Harmony Books; 1993.

Coleman, Donald A., M.D., Nancy Szeman, R.D., C.D.E.; *The Top 100 International Low-Fat Recipes;* Time-Life Books, Inc.; 1996.

The Complete German Commission E Monographs, Therapeutic Guide to Herbal Medicines; Senior Editor, Mark Blumenthal; American Botanical Council; 1998.

Cranton, Elmore, M.D., Arlene Brecher; *Bypassing Bypass, The New Technique of Chelation Therapy;* 1990; 2d edition, Stein & Day; 1984.

Crayhon, Robert, M.S.; *The Carnitine Miracle;* Evans; 1998.

Dacher, Elliott S., M.D.; *Psychoneuroimmunology The New Mind/Body Healing Program;* Paragon House; 1991.

D'Adamo, Peter J., M.D., Catherine Whitney; *Four Blood Types, Four Diets, Eat Right for Your Type, The Invidualized Diet Solution to Staying Healthy, Living Longer and Achieving Your Ideal Weight;* Putnam; 1996.

Danbrot, Margaret; *The New Cabbage Soup Diet;* Lynn Sanberg, Book Associates; 1997.

Danniston, Denise, Peter McWilliams; *The Transcendental Meditation Book;* Warner Books; 1975.

Eades, Michael R., M.D., Mary Dan Eades, M.D.; *Protein Power;* Bantam Books; 1996.

Fritzweiss, Rudolph, M.D.; *Herbal Medicine;* Beaconsfield Publishers, Ltd.; 1988; 4th edition; 1996.

Goldberg, Burton, Editors of Alternative Medicine Digest; *Alternative Medicine Guide to Heart Disease;* Future Medicine Publishing; 1998.

Goldstrich, Joe D., M.D., F.A.C.C.; *The Cardiologist's Painless Prescription for a Healthy Heart and a Longer Life;* 9-Heart-9 Publishing; 1994.

Josephson, Mark E., M.D.; *Clinical Cardiac Electrophysiology;* Lea and Febiger; 1993.

Kabat-Zinn, John, Ph.D.; *Full Catastrophe Living;* Dell; 1990.

Kirschmann, Gayla J., John D. Kirschmann; *Nutrition Almanac;* McGraw-Hill; 1996.

Klein, Alan; *The Healing Power of Humor;* Jeremy P. Tarcher/Putnam; 1989.

Lipetz, Philip, Monika Pichler; *Naturally Slim and Powerful;* Andrews McMeel, a Universal Press Syndicated Co.; 1997.

McArdle, William, Frank Katch, Victor Katch; *Exercise Physiology, Energy, Nutrition and Human Performance;* Williams Wilkins; 1996.

McCulley, Kilmer S., M.D.; *The Homocysteine Revolution;* Keats Publishing; 1997.

Mabberley, D. J.; *The Plant Book;* Cambridge University Press; 1997.

Mabey, Richard; *The New Age Herbalist;* Simon & Schuster; 1988.

Mills, Simon Y.; *The Essential Book of Herbal Medicine;* Penguin; 1991.

Murray, Michael T., N.D.; *Encyclopedia of Nutritional Supplements;* Prima Publishing; 1996.

Murray, Michael T., N.D.; *The Healing Power of Herbs;* Prima Publishing; 1992; 2d edition; 1995.

Murray, Michael T., N.D.; *Heart Disease and High Blood Pressure, How*

You Can Benefit from Diet, Vitamins, Minerals, Herbs, Exercise And Other Natural Methods; Prima Publishing; 1997.

Murray, Michael T., N.D.; *Natural Alternatives to Over the Counter and Prescription Drugs;* William Morrow; 1994.

Murray, Michael T., N.D., Joseph Pizzorno, N.D.; *Encyclopedia of Natural Medicine;* Prima Publishing; 1991.

Ornish, Dean, M.D.; *Dr. Dean Ornish's Program for Reversing Heart Disease;* Ballantine Books; 1990.

Ornish, Dean, M.D.; *Love and Survival;* HarperCollins; 1997.

Ortiz, Elizabeth Lambert; *The Encyclopedia of Herbs, Spices and Flavorings;* Dorling Kindersley; 1992.

Peckenpaugh, Nancy J., Charlotte M. Polman; *Nutrition, Essentials and Diet Therapy;* Saunders; 1995.

Pedersen, Mark; *Nutritional Herbology, A Reference Guide to Herbs;* Wendell W. Wittman, 1994.

Petersdorf, Adam, Brawnwal, Martin Isselbacher, Wilson; *Harrison's Principles of Internal Medicine;* McGraw-Hill, Inc., 10th edition, 1983.

Pollock, Michael L., Ph.D., Jack Wilmore, Ph.D.; *Exercise in Health and Disease;* Saunders; 1990.

Price, Shirley, Len Price; *Aromatherapy for Health Professionals;* Churchill Livingstone Press; 1995.

Pritikin, Nathan; *The Pritikin Program for Diet and Exercise;* Bantam; 1987 (reissue).

Pritikin, Robert; *The Pritikin Weight Loss Breakthrough;* Dutton; 1998.

Rosenfeld, Isadore, M.D.; *Dr. Rosenfeld's Guide to Alternative Medicine;* Random House; 1996.

Rothfeld, Glenn S., M.D., Suzanne Luvert; *Natural Medicine for Heart Disease, The Best Alternative Methods for Prevention and Treatment;* Rodale Press; 1996.

Sachs, Judith; *Natural Medicine for Heart Disease;* Dell; 1996.

Schlant, Robert C., Wayne R. Alexander; *Hurst's: The Heart;* McGraw Hill, Inc., 4th edition, 1994.

Sears, Barry, Ph.D., with Bill Lawrence; *The Zone;* Regan Books; 1995.

Selye, Hans; *Stress Without Distress;* Cygnet Press; 1974.

Shute, Evan V., F.R.S.C.(C); *The Heart and Vitamin E;* Keats Publishing; 1956; most recent edition; 1977.

Sinatra, Steven T., M.D.; *Heartbreak and Heart Disease;* Keats Publishing; 1996.

Skinner, James S.; *Exercise Testing and Exercise Prescription for Special Cases;* Lea and Febiger; 1993.

Strauss, Richard H., M.D., Editor; *Sports Medicine;* Saunders; 1991.

Tyler, Varoe, Ph.D.; *The Honest Herbal;* Pharmaceutical Products Press; 1982; 3d edition; 1993.

Ward, David E., M.D., A. John Camm, M.D.; *Clinical Electrophysiology of the Heart;* Edward Arnold; 1987.

Weil, Andrew, M.D.; *Health and Healing;* Houghton Mifflin; 1983; most recent edition; 1995.

Weil, Andrew, M.D.; *Spontaneous Healing;* Fawcett Columbine; 1995.

Wildwood, Chrissie; *Encyclopedia of Aromatherapy;* Healing Arts Press; 1996.

Wyngaarden, Smith; *Cecil Textbook of Medicine;* Saunders; 1987.

Zipes, Douglas, José Jalife; *Cardiac Electrophysiology from Cell to Bedside;* Saunders; 1990.

Resource Guide

The following is a list of recommended supplement and resource companies that the reader may contact for information about products for heart and total body health.

Boiron USA
6 Campus Drive, Building A
Newtown Square, PA 19073
1-800-258-8823

Carlson Laboratories
15 College Drive
Arlington Heights, IL 60004
1-800-323-4141

Crown Prince
18581 Railroad Street
City of Industry, CA 91748
1-800-255-5063

Dr. Hauschka Skin Care
59-C North Street
Hatfield, MA 01038
1-800-247-9907

Enzymatic Therapy
825 Challenger Drive
Green Bay, WI 54311
1-800-558-7372

Flora
P.O. Box 73, 805 E. Badger Road
Lynden, WA 98264
1-800-498-3610

Frey Vineyards
14000 Tomki Road
Redwood Valley, CA 95470
1-800-760-3739

Gaia Herbs
108 Island Ford Road
Brevard, NC 28712
1-800-831-7780

Goldmine Natural Food Company
1-800-475-3663
http://www.goldminenaturalfood.com

Natrol®
20731 Marilla Street
Chatsworth, CA 91311
1-800-326-1520

Nature's Herbs®
600 E. Quality Drive
American Fork, Utah 84003
1-800-437-2257

N.E.E.D.S
Nutritional, Ecological & Environmental Delivery System
1-800-634-1380
http://www.needs4u.com

Solaray
1500 Kearns Blvd., Ste. B-200
Park City, UT 84060
1-800-683-9640

Solgar Vitamin & Herb
500 Willow Tree Road
Leonia, NJ 07605
1-800-645-2246

Wakunaga of America Co., Ltd.
23501 Madero
Mission Viejo, CA 92691
1-800-421-2998

Bath Oils for Stress

Available from the following company:

Dr. Hauschka Skin Care
Pine, Lemon, and Lavender bath oils

COQ10

Available from the following companies:

Carlson®
PRODUCT NAME: CO-Q10
Available in 10 mg, 30 mg, 50 mg, 100 mg, and 200 mg soft gels.

Enzymatic Therapy
PRODUCT NAME: COQ10
Available in 50 mg soft gels.

Coleus Forskohii

Available from the following company:

Enzymatic Therapy
PRODUCT NAME: Coleus Forskohlii Extract
Each capsule contains 50 mg Coleus Forskohlii Extract,
standardized to contain a minimum of 18% forskolin (9 mg per capsule).

Vitamin E—100% Natural-Source

Available from the following company:

Carlson®
PRODUCT NAME: Key-E® Chewable Tablets
Natural-source Vitamin E in 100 i.u., 200 i.u., and 400 i.u. chewable
tablets.

PRODUCT NAME: Key-E® Kaps
Natural-source Vitamin E in 200–400 i.u. capsules.

PRODUCT NAME: E-Gems®
Contains concentrated natural-source Vitamin E oil.
Available in soft gels in eight different strengths, from 30 i.u. to 1200 i.u.

PRODUCT NAME: E-Gems Plus
Contains natural-source Vitamin E derived from soybean oil supplying

alpha tocopherol plus other tocopherols. Available in 200 i.u., 400 i.u., and 800 i.u. soft gels

PRODUCT NAME: d-Alpha Gems™
Contains natural-source Vitamin E in the highest concentration possible (1360 i.u. per gram). Available in 400 i.u. soft gels.

PRODUCT NAME: E-Sel
Contains 400 i.u. natural-source Vitamin E and 100 mcg organic Selenium in soft gels.

Natural Vitamin E for the skin

Available from the following company:

Carlson®
PRODUCT NAME: E-Gem® Oil Drops
Each drop contains 10 i.u. of Vitamin E derived from soybean oil.
Apply externally to aid and soften the skin.

PRODUCT NAME: Key-E® Spray
Each 3 seconds of spray on the skin provides approximately 30 i.u. of Natural-Source Vitamin E.

Essential Fatty Acids/Fish Oils

Available from the following companies:

Carlson®
PRODUCT NAME: Super Omega-3 Fish Oils
Each soft gel contains 330 mg EPA, 220 mg DHA and 40 mg other omega-3 fatty acids.

PRODUCT NAME: Super DHA™
Each soft gel contains 500 mg DHA and 200 mg EPA.

Solgar
PRODUCT NAME: Mega Max EPA
Contains 750 mg EPA/DHA per two soft gels.

Fish—high in essential fatty acids

Canned fish available from the following company:

Crown Prince, Inc.
PRODUCT NAMES: Brisling Sardines in Pure Olive Oil, Brisling Sardines in Water, Pink Salmon, Albacore Tuna in Spring Water and Albacore Tuna in Water—Low Sodium.

Flax Oil

Available from the following company:

Flora
PRODUCT NAME: Flax Oil
Contains certified organic flax oil, bottled in opaque glass, complete with pressing date.

Flax Seeds

Available from the following company:

Flora
PRODUCT NAME: Golden Flax Seed
Certified organic and nitrogen flushed when bottled to ensure freshness.

Garlic Supplements

Available from the following companies:

Enzymatic Therapy©
PRODUCT NAME: Garlinase 4000®
Each enteric-coated tablet contains 4,000 mg of fresh garlic

Wakunaga
PRODUCT NAME: Kyolic® Aged Garlic Extract™
Organically grown, 100% odorless

Ginkgo Biloba

Available from the following companies:

Carlson®
PRODUCT NAME: Ginkgo Biloba plus L-Glutamine
Contains 40 mg Ginkgo Biloba Extract and 200 mg L-Glutamine in soft gel form.

Solaray
PRODUCT NAME: Ginkgo Biloba Extract
Each capsule contains 60 mg Ginkgo biloba extract with a guaranteed potency of 14.4 mg (24%) ginkgoflavoglycosides and 3.6 mg (6%) terpene lactones.

PRODUCT NAME: Ginkgo Phytosome®
Each capsule contains 180 mg Ginkgo Phytosome (24% ginkgoflavoglycoside Ginkgo biloba extract bound to phosphatidyl choline). *Phytosome is a registered trademark of Idena S.P.A.

Hawthorn

Available from the following company:

Gaia Herbs
PRODUCT NAME: Hawthorn Supreme
Hawthorn Berry Extract made from Hawthorn berries, flowers and leaves in a 2.5:1 weight-to-volume ratio. Suggested dosage: 2 dropperfuls taken in a small amount of warm water.

Kava Kava

Available from the following companies:

Carlson®
PRODUCT NAME: Kava
Standardized potency Kava extract in 150 mg soft gels.

Natrol®
PRODUCT NAME: Kavatrol®
Standardized potency Kava extract in capsules and tablets.

Mail Order

Available from the following companies:

Goldmine Natural Food Company
Organic grains, beans and seeds, soy products, and Japanese green teas.

N.E.E.D.S
Supplements and vitamins, health and beauty aids, and books

Multivitamin/Mineral Formulation for Heart Health

Available from the following company:

Carlson®
PRODUCT NAME: Heartbeat Elite™
An outstanding formula based on scientific studies and research, Heartbeat Elite™ provides more than 25 nutrients to support a healthy cardiovascular system. Suitable for vegetarians. Formulated by Dr. Seth Baum. Available in tablets.

Olive Oil

Available from the following company:

Flora
PRODUCT NAME: Extra Virgin Oilve Oil
Certified organic, bottled in opaque glass, complete with pressing date.

Oscillococcinum

Available from the following company:

Boiron
Homeopathic flu medicine available in boxes of three unit dose tubes (one treatment regimen) or six unit does tubes (two treatment regimens).

Pygeum

Available from the following companies:

Enzymatic Therapy
PRODUCT NAME: Nettle & Pygeum with Pumpkin
Each capsule contains 300 mg Nettle Root Extract, 175 mg Pumpkin Seed Oil and 25 mg Pygeum Africanum Extract.

Solaray
PRODUCT NAME: Pygeum Africanum Extract
Each capsule contains 50 mg Pygeum africanum bark extract with a guaranteed potency of 6.5 mg (13%) total sterols.

Saw Palmetto

Available from the following companies:

Enzymatic Therapy:
PRODUCT NAME: Saw Palmetto Complex
Each capsule contains 80 mg Saw Palmetto Extract, 40 mg Pumpkin Seed Oil Extract, 10 mg Pygeum Africanum Extract, and 5 mg Bearberry Extract

Solaray
PRODUCT NAME: Saw Palmetto Berry Extract
Each perlecap (soft gel) contains 160 mg Saw Palmetto berry extract with a guaranteed potency of 136 mg (85%) fatty acids and sterols minimum.

Selenium

Available from the following companies:

Carlson®
PRODUCT NAME: Selenium
Contains Selenium organically bound to yeast.
Available in 50 mcg tablets or 150 mcg capsules.

PRODUCT NAME: Selenium
Contains Selenium organically bound to Methionine. Yeast-free.
Available in 200 mcg capsules and tablets.

Natrol®
PRODUCT NAME: Selenium 200 Mcg
Available in 200 mcg tablets.

Solgar
PRODUCT NAME: Seleno Precise™
Selenium available in 50 mcg, 100 mcg, and 200 mcg tablets.

Slippery Elm Bark

Available from the following company:

Nature's Herbs®
PRODUCT NAME: Slippery Elm
Each gelatin capsule contains 340 mg Wild Countryside Slippery Elm
Inner Bark

Wine

Available from the following company:

Frey Vineyards
Organic wines with no sulfites added.

Listed below are pharmaceutical companies whose drugs Dr. Baum
uses in his practice:

Boehringer Ingelheim Pharmaceuticals, Inc.
900 Ridgebury Road
Ridgefield, CT 06877
1-800-542-6257
NAME OF DRUG: Catapres

Ciba Geneva Pharmaceuticals
556 Morris Avenue
Summit, NJ 07901
1-800-526-0175
NAME OF DRUG: Lopressor

DuPont
Chestnut Run Plaza
Hickory Run
Wilmington, DE 19880
302-995-5000
NAME OF DRUG: Coumadin

Glaxco Wellcome
5 Moor Drive
Research Triangle Park, NC 27709
919-483-2100
NAME OF DRUG: Lanoxin/Digoxin

Hoechst Marion Roussel
10235 Marion Park Drive
Kansas City, MO 64134
1-800-321-0855
NAMES OF DRUGS: Cardizem, Lasix

Key Pharmaceuticals, Inc.
Galloping Hill Road
Kenilworth, NJ 07033
1-800-222-7579
NAMES OF DRUGS: Imdur, Nitro-Dur

Kos Pharmaceuticals
1001 Brickell Bay Road
Miami, FL 33131
1-800-722-4567
NAME OF DRUG: Niaspan

Medeva
P.O. Box 1740
Rochester, NY 14603
716-274-5300
NAME OF DRUG: Zaroxolyn

Merck and Co.
P.O. Box 4
West Point, PA 19486
1-800-737-2088
NAMES OF DRUGS: Cozaar, Hyzaar, Mevacor, Vasotec

Mylan Pharmaceutical
781 Chestnut Ridge Road
Morgantown, WV 26504
304-599-2595
NAME OF DRUG: Captopril

Pfizer, Inc.
235 East 42nd Street
New York, NY 10017
1-800-879-3477
NAMES OF DRUGS: Cardura, Lipitor, Norvasc, Procardia

Smithkline Beecham Pharmaceuticals
One Franklin Plaza
Philadelphia, PA 19101
1-800-366-8906
NAME OF DRUG: Coreg

Zeneca Labs
Wilmington, DE 19850
302-886-8000
NAME OF DRUG: Tenormin

Manufacturers of Medical Equipment

ACS
3200 Lakeside Drive
P.O. Box 58167
Santa Clara, CA 95052-8167
1-800-227-9902
(angioplasty balloons and stents)

Guidant Corporation
4100 Hamline Ave. N.
Saint Paul, MN 55112-5798
1-800-CARDIAC
(pacemakers and defibrillators)

Scimed
1 Scimed Place
Maple Grove, MN 55311
612-494-1700
(angioplasty balloons and rotablators)

Organizations and Governmental Agencies

American College of Advancement of Medicine (ACAM)
23121 Verduga Drive, Suite 204
Laguna Hills, CA 92653
1-800-532-3688

American Heart Association
300 NE Spanish River Blvd
Boca Raton, FL 33431
1-800-242-8721

American College of Cardiology
9111 Old Georgetown Road
Bethesda, MD 20814
1-800-253-4363

American Medical Association
515 N. State Street
Chicago, IL 60610
1-800-621-8335

Bastyr University
14500 Juanita Drive NE
Bothwell, WA 98011
425-602-3003

Center for Complementary and Alternative Medicine
9000 Rockville Pike
Building 31 5B38
Bethesda, MD 20814
888-644-6226

Friends of Chelation
255 N. El Cielo Road, Suite 670
Palm Springs, CA 92262
760-776-9338

National Cholesterol Education Program
9000 Rockville Pike
Bldg 31, Room 4A16
Bethesda, MD 20814
301-496-4000

National Coalition of Certified Aromatherapist and Aromatology
    of Practioners
P.O. Box 835025
Miami, FL 33283
305-595-4776

National Institues of Health
9000 Rockville Pike
Bethesda, MD 20814
301-496-4000

Websites

AMERICAN MEDICAL ASSOCIATION
www.ama-assn.org

ASK DR. WEIL
cgi.pathfinder.comb/drweil

BAUM CENTER FOR INTEGRA-
TIVE HEART CARE
www.baumheartctr.com

CENTERS FOR DISEASE
CONTROL
www.cdc.gov

HEALTHY WAY
www.sympatico.ca/healthyway

HERBAL REFERENCE LIBRARY
www.all-natural.com
www.all-natural.com/
    herbindx.html

HOMEOPATHIC EDUCATIONAL
SERVICES
www.homeopathic.com

NATIONAL INSTITUTE OF
AYURVEDIC MEDICINE
www.niam.com

NATIONAL INSTITUTES OF
HEALTH
www.nih.gov

QI: THE JOURNAL OF TRADI-
TIONAL EASTERN HEALTH
AND FITNESS
www.qi-journal.com

THRIVE
www.thriveonline.com

TUFTS UNIVERSITY'S NUTRITION
NAVIGATOR
www.navigator.tufts.edu

YOGAAAHHH
www2.gdi.net/-mjm/asana.htm

Index

A-betalipoproteinemia, 51
A-Strand study, 217
ablation catheter, 143
ACE inhibitors, 65, 92, 93, 115–16,
    119, 125, 126
Adenosine, 27
adrenaline, 223, 224
aerobic training, 216–18
African Americans: idiopathic di-
    lated cardiomyopathy in men,
    108; salt sensitivity in, 186
afterload reducing agents, 126
agglutination, 162
aging process, coronary artery dis-
    ease and the, 35–36, 37
alcohol, 52, 175
alcohol-related cardiomyopathy,
    110–11
alkaloids, 199
allicin, 203
allopathic medicine, 1–2
aloe leaf, 200, 214
alpha lipoic acid, 43, 50, 59, 84,
    172, 191–92
alpha tocopherol, 175
alternative medicine practitioners,
    237–38
American College of Advancement
    of Medicine (ACAM), 100
American Heart Association, 28
amino acids, 99, 100, 157, 188

ammonium salts, 45–46
anaerobic training, 216, 218–20
anger, 226–27
"anger recall" study, 226
angina: aortic stenosis, 129; in Type
    A behavior patterns, 58; unstable,
    11, 80–85
angina pectoris, 63–65
angiograms, 2–3, 4, 29–30, 84, 119
angioplasty, 1, 4, 71–74, 83, 87, 90,
    91, 119
Angioplasty Compared to Medicine
    (ACME) trial, 71
angiotensin converting enzyme in-
    hibitors (ACE inhibitors), 65, 92,
    93, 115–16, 119, 125, 126
ankle-branchial indices, 24
antibiotics, 123, 137, 138
anticoagulation, 133–35
antidepressants, 159
antioxidants, 50, 172–73, 208; low
    levels of, 36, 38, 58–59; for treat-
    ing angina pectoris, 70, 71; for
    treating unstable angina, 84
antiplatelet agents, 75, 83
aortic regurgitation, 130–31
aortic root disease, 131
aortic sclerosis, 22
aortic stenosis, 128–30
aortic valve disease, 128
aortocoronary bypass (ACB), 76–80

apical hypertrophic cardiomyopathy, 112
arachidonic acid, 165
arginine, 99, 100
aromatherapy, 229–30
aromatic herbs, 197, 198, 213
arrhythmias, 190
arthritis, 193
asparagus root, 200, 214
aspirin, 24, 199; for angina pectoris, 64–65, 66, 68; for heart attacks, 87, 89, 92, 94; for TIAs, 127; for unstable angina, 82
asthma, 67
astringent herbs, 197, 198–99, 214
atenolol, 148
atherosclerosis, 4, 88, 165, 204
Atkins diet, 162–63
Atkins, Robert, 151, 165
atrial fibrillation, 23, 99, 117, 123, 135, 141, 264–66
atrioventricular block, 129
atrioventricular node (A-V node), 15–16, 141
atrioventricular valves, 13
Ayurvedic medicine, 237

backward failure, 104
backward right heart failure, 105
bacterial endocarditis, 138
Balch, James F., 167
Balch, Phyllis A., 167
balloon angioplasty, 71, 72
balloon mitral valvuloplasty, 124, 130
Barlow syndrome, 127
Batista operation, 115, 118
Baum Center for Integrative Heart Care, 238
benign prostatic hypertrophy (BPH), 211, 212
Benson, Herbert, 231
beta agonists, 117
beta blockers: for angina pectoris, 65, 67, 68, 69; as cause for high triglycerides, 52; coenzyme Q-10 and, 191; for fainting, 148; for heart attacks, 87, 89, 92, 93; for heart failure, 106, 112, 115, 117; for hypertrophic cardiomyopathy, 112; for mitral stenosis, 123; for mitral valve prolapse, 127; for unstable angina, 82
beta carotene, 169, 175
betaine, 98
bilberry, 209–10
bile acid sequestrants, 45–46
bioflavonoids, 207, 208, 209
bitter herbs, 197, 199, 214
black tea, 208
Blake, William, 232
blood, 36; blood factors, 59–61; mitral stenosis, 122
blood clots, 23; in heart attacks, 88, 95; in valvular heart disease, 123–24, 127, 134, 135
blood pressure, 5–6; complications and heart attacks, 95; helpful supplements for high, 190; hypertension (high blood pressure), 19, 23, 36, 37, 54–55; systolic, 14
blood thinners: blood clots and, 23; for heart attacks, 90, 95; medications for chronic stable angina pectoris, 65; medications for unstable angina, 82; for valvular disease, 123, 127, 134
blood type, dietary recommendations according to, 151, 160–62
bradycardias, 253–59
Braunwald, Eugene, 65
bromelain, 70, 71
Bruce protocol, 25
bruits, 18, 24
bypass grafting, 1, 4, 76–80
bypass tracts, 141, 146, 262

cabbage soup diet, 166
caffeine, 168
calcium, 56, 100, 170, 185–86
calcium carbonate, 186
calcium channel blockers: for heart attacks, 87, 89; magnesium as

natural, 183; medications for angina pectoris, 65, 68–70; for mitral regurgitation, 125
calcium citrate, 186
calcium deposits, 28
calcium gluconate, 186
Cambridge Heart Antioxidant Study (CHAOS), 176
Canadian Coronary Atherosclerosis Intervention Trial (CCAIT), 42
cancer, 11
captopril, 115, 116
carbohydrates, 152–54, 159
Cardiac Arrhythmia Suppression Trial (CAST), 257, 259
cardiac beta receptors, 106
cardiac catheterization, 2–3, 29–30
cardiac conditions, supplements that help manage, 190
cardiac rehabilitation, 95
cardiac valve prostheses, 132–36
cardiogenic shock, 94, 95
Cardiolite, 28
cardiomyopathies, 108–13, 117
cardiovascular health, herbs promoting, 202–13
Carnitine Miracle, The (Crayhon), 189
carotenoids, 175
carotid sinus massage, 145
carotid ultrasound, 23–24
cascara, 199, 214
catheters, 3, 141–43
cayenne pepper, 47, 182, 206
cerebrovascular disease, 54
chelation therapy, 100–101
children: causes of heart failure in, 112, 113; cholesterol screening for, 50; with congenital long QT syndrome, 268–69; with hypertrophic cardiomyopathy, 112; lesions in, 35
Chinese restaurant syndrome, 179
cholesterol, 50–53; culinary herbs and high, 47; egg's cholesterol content, 167–68; garlic in lowering, 204; low cholesterol levels,

51; vitamin C in lowering, 177; vitamins and supplements for modifying, 42–43. *See also* hypercholesterolemia (high cholesterol)
cholesterol-lowering medications, 41, 42, 43–44, 45–50, 64
cholesterol-lowering studies, 40–45
cholesterol-lowering supplements, 17, 39, 42–43, 181–83
cholesterol-lowering therapy, 50–51
cholestipol, 45
cholestyramine, 41, 42, 43, 45
choline, 43, 180, 181
chordae tendineae, 124, 125
chromium, 57, 84, 170, 181
chronic stable angina pectoris, 63–65, 76, 81
chylomicrons, 39
circulatory system, the heart and, 12, 104
citrate, 186
citrus bioflavonoids, 208
claudication, 184, 188, 190
clofibrate, 41
clots. *See* blood clots
clotting: cardiac valve prostheses and, 133–35; elevated levels of clotting factors, 39; garlic's anti-blood-clotting effects, 204; helpful supplements for clotting problems, 190; nitroglycerine's anticlotting effects, 66
cobalamin, 179–80
coenzyme Q-10, 57, 59, 172, 189, 191; for angina pectoris, 70, 71; for heart attacks, 98, 100; for heart failure, 106–7, 119, 137; L-carnitine and, 188; for lowering high blood pressure, 54, 56; magnesium and, 184; for unstable angina, 84; for valvular heart disease, 128, 131, 136, 137
coffee consumption, 168
coleus, 54, 56, 204–5
collagen, 173, 186
Collins, Michael, 29, 30

color flow Doppler, 22
Complete German Commission E Monographs (Blumenthal), 202–3
complex carbohydrates, 152, 153
complex lesions, 35
congenital long QT syndromes, 268–69
congestive heart failure, 94, 95, 99, 103; acute, 117; aortic stenosis, 129, 130; body's response to heart failure, 105–7; heart muscle diseases, 108–13; helpful supplements for, 190; treating, 114–19; what happens in heart failure?, 103–5
CONSENSUS trial, 116
copper, 84, 100, 170, 186–87
cor bovinum, 130
coronary arteries, 14–15
coronary artery bypass grafting (CABG), 1, 4, 76–80
coronary artery disease, 17, 20, 33–35, 49; blood factors, 59–61; cholesterol, 50–53; cholesterol-lowering medications, 45–50; diabetes, 55–57; hypertension, 54–55; low levels of antioxidants, 58–59; obesity, 57; observational studies, 40–45; physical inactivity, 57–58; risk factors for, 35–36, 37–39; tobacco, 53–54; Type A behavior pattern, 58
Coronary Artery Drug Project study, 49
Coronary Artery Surgical Study (CASS), 77–78
coronary care unit (CCU), 87, 91–92
Coronary Drug Project, 42
Coumadin (blood thinner), 23, 65, 95, 123, 127, 133, 134
Cozaar, 116
Crayhon, Robert, 189
crescendo angina, 80
Cretan diet, 164
Crohn's disease, 131

D'Adamo, Peter J., 151, 160–62
Danbrodt, Margaret, 166
deglycyrrhizinated licorice (DGL), 212–13
delayed-onset muscle soreness (DOMS), 222
dental cleaning, 137–38
depression, 228
diabetes, 55–57; aortic stenosis and, 128; as cause for high triglycerides, 52, 55; dilated cardiomyopathy and, 111; as risk factor for coronary heart disease, 36, 37
diabetic neuropathies, 192
diabetic retinopathy, 56
diastole, 13, 105, 124
diet, balanced, 7, 151–52; carbohydrates, 152–54; fat, 154–57; popular diets, 158–69; protein, 157–58. *See also* food
digitalis, 114, 115
Digoxin, 114, 115, 119, 123, 126, 202
dilated cardiomyopathy (DCM), 108–12
diltiazem, 68, 69–70
Diovan, 116
directional coronary atherectomy (DCA), 72
disaccharides, 153
diuretics, 52, 114, 119, 123, 126
Dobutamine, 27–28, 118
dolomite, 186
down regulation of cardiac beta receptors, 106
Dressler's syndrome, 94
dried standardized herbs, 201–2
drugs. *See* medications
duration, exercise, 216

Eat Right for Your Type (D'Adamo), 160–62
echinacea, 138
echocardiogram (ECHO), 22, 23, 191; in diagnosing aortic regurgitation, 131; in diagnosing aortic stenosis, 130; in diagnosing mi-

tral valve prolapse, 127; sedentary stress tests and echocardiography, 27–28

eggs, 167–68

eicosanoids, 165

elastin, 186

electrocardiogram (ECG or EKG), 19–20, 21, 23, 26

electrolytes, 114

electrophysiology, 139; basic electrophysiology study, 140–46; electrical abnormalities of the heart, 253–69; electrical misfires of the heart, 146–49

emboli (blood clots), 123–24, 127, 135

empty heart syndrome, 148

enalapril, 115, 116

Encyclopedia of Nutritional Supplements, The (Murray), 172

endocarditis prophylaxis, 129

endothelial-derived relaxing factor (EDRF), 34

endurance, muscular, 219

epinephrine, 89, 223, 231

erythromycin, 47

essential fatty acids, 43, 155, 192–93; for anticoagulation, 134; L-carnitine and, 188; magnesium and, 184

estrogen replacement therapy (ERT), 48–50, 52

European Cooperative Surgical Study (ECSS), 77–78

event recorders, 21

Excimer laser, 73

exercise, 2, 7, 28, 215–16; aerobic, 30; aerobic training, 216– 18; fainting and, 129; flexibility, 216, 221–22; heart attack patients and, 97, 98; nonexercise stress test, 27; physical inactivity, 38, 57–58; resistance or weight training, 216, 218–20

Factor 7, 59

fainting: aortic stenosis, 129; chil-
dren with congenital long QT syndrome, 268–69; children with hypertrophic cardiomyopathy, 112; common types of, 148–49; neurally mediated syncope, 147–48

fats: dietary, 154–57, 158; lipids, 34, 35, 36; serum lipids, 188–89, 228. *See also* triglycerides

feverfew, 212

fiber: complex carbohydrates with high fiber content, 153; dietary, 54, 55; soluble and insoluble, 47, 153–54, 182; supplements, 57; water-soluble fibers and lower cholesterol, 39

fibric acid derivatives, 48, 49

fibrinogen, 36, 59–60, 178, 193

"fight or flight" response, 9, 105–6, 223

fish oils, 52, 55, 192

flavonoids, 207–9

flexibility training, 216, 221–22

Florinef, 148

flushing effects, niacin and its, 178

folic acid, 98, 100, 169, 178–79

food: cold water fish, 52, 55, 192; diet for blood pressure reduction, 54–55; diet and triglycerides, 52; dietary adjustments for heart attack patients, 98; foods for cardiovascular health, 153, 156–57; foods containing calcium, 185; foods containing essential fatty acids, 192; foods containing potassium, 187; grapefruit, 209; malnutrition and alcohol abuse, 111; onions, 56; sources of important nutrients, 169–70; vegetables containing vitamin C, 177

forward failure, 104

forward right heart failure, 105

founder effect, 161

Framingham Heart Study: coronary heart disease, 35–36; obesity, 57;

Framingham Heart Study (*cont.*)
  smoking, 53; Type A behavior
  pattern, 58, 226
free radicals, 60–61, 100, 172–73,
  176
"freeze frame" technique, 10, 30,
  232–33
frequency, exercise, 216
Friedman, Meyer, 226
fructose, 152

galactose, 152, 153
gamma camera, 26
garlic: for anticoagulation, 134; for
  bacterial endocarditis, 138; cardiovascular advantages of, 203–4;
  for heart attacks, 98, 99; for lowering cholesterol, 17, 39, 47, 182;
  for lowering high blood pressure,
  56
gastroesophageal reflux, 18
Gemifibrozil, 41, 48, 59
German E Commission, 199, 202–3,
  204, 205, 209, 211
ginger, fresh, 56
gingival hyperplasia, 69
ginkgo biloba, 134, 184, 188, 205–6
ginseng, 182
gluconate, 186
glucose, 56, 152, 153
glutathione peroxidase, 172, 187
glycoprotein IIB/IIIA platelet inhibitors, 83
grapefruit, 209
grapeseed extract, 43, 50, 59, 84
green tea, 208
Greenland Eskimos, study of the,
  52
Grunzig, Andreas, 71
guar gum, 47, 99, 100, 154
gugulipid, 39, 47, 98, 99, 182,
  206–7

hawthorn, 202–3, 207; for angina
  pectoris, 70, 71; for heart attacks,
  98, 100; for heart failure, 107; for
  lowering high blood pressure, 54,
  56; for valvular heart disease,
  126, 131, 136, 137
HDL. *See* high density lipoproteins
  (HDL, "good" cholesterol)
Healing Power of Herbs, The (Murray), 211–12
Healing Power of Humor, The (Klein),
  229
health food stores, 171
heart attacks (myocardial infarctions), 27, 33, 87–88, 237–38;
  acute myocardial infarction, 63,
  80; age and, 35; causes of, 88;
  complications of, 93–95; diagnosis and treatment of, 89– 93; life
  style modifications after a heart
  attack, 97–98; lowering mortality
  from, 92; natural methods of
  treating heart attack patients,
  96–101, 188, 190; primary treatment of, 91; secondary treatment
  of, 92
heart block, 255–56
heart failure. *See* congestive heart
  failure
heart murmurs, 19, 22, 138
heart muscle diseases, 108–13
heart rhythm disturbances: abnormal heart rhythms and their
  treatments, 253–69; in congestive
  heart failure, 117, 118; electrophysiology, 139–49; in heart attack victims, 94, 95; stress and,
  227; *torsade de pointes,* 184; in
  valvular heart disease, 127, 129
heart tests, 17–31
heart, the, 9–16, 33–34, 104–5; electrical abnormalities of, 253–69;
  electrical circuitry, 15–16, 144;
  resting heart rate, 67
heart transplants, 118
heart valve abnormalities, 22
heart valves, 122
heartburn, 18
Helsinki Heart Study, 41
hemoptysis, 122
heparin, 82, 83, 89

herbs, 195–97, 200–202; for angina pectoris, 70, 71; for aortic regurgitation, 131; aromatic, 197, 198, 213; astringent, 197, 198–99, 214; bitter, 197, 199, 214; of cardiovascular appeal, 202–13; culinary herbs and high cholesterol, 47; for heart attacks, 98; helpful in managing medical ailments, 213–14; for hypertension, 54; mucilaginous, 197, 199–200, 214; nutritive, 197, 200, 214

high blood pressure. *See* blood pressure; hypertension (high blood pressure)

high density lipoproteins (HDL, "good" cholesterol), 39; aerobic training and, 217; beta blockers and, 67; cholesterol-lowering medications and, 45, 46, 48; diabetes, 55; garlic and increase in, 204; gugulipid and increase in, 206; omega-3 fatty acids and increase in, 52; vitamin C and increase in, 177

histidine, 157

HMG-CoA reductase inhibitors (statins), 46, 47–48, 49, 191

Holter monitors, 21

homocysteine, 36, 38, 59, 60, 98, 179

homograft valves, 135

hypercholesterolemia (high cholesterol), 36, 39, 206; as risk factor for coronary heart disease, 36, 37; studies, 40–41, 45

hyperinsulinemia, 162, 165

hyperlipidemia, 167

hypertension (high blood pressure), 19, 23, 36, 37, 54–55; calcium channel blockers for managing, 70; helpful supplements for, 56, 190

hypertriglyceridemia, 45, 51

hypertrophic cardiomyopathy (HCM), 108, 109, 112–13

hypertrophy, 106

hypothyroidism, 52, 254

idiopathic dilated cardiomyopathy (IDCM), 108–10

imaging centers, 22

immunosuppressive drugs, 118

implantable cardioverter defibrillators (ICDs), 112, 267

inositol hexaniacinate, 178

inotropy, 67, 69, 70, 118, 202, 204

insulin, 57, 90, 159, 203

integrative health care, birth of, 1–8

integrative heart care, future of, 235–39

intensity, exercise, 216

intermediate density lipoproteins (IDL), 39

intermittent claudication, 184

interventional cardiology, 70–76

interventional trials, 40–42, 52, 58, 226

intra-aortic balloon pump (IABP), 80

intracardiac electrogram, 143

intuitive medicine, 10–11

iron, 59, 60–61, 100, 170

ischemia, 27, 28; silent ischemia, 64, 228

ISIS 4, 97

isolation, social, 228

isoleucine, 157

isometric exercise, 219–20

Isordil, 115, 116

isotonic training, 220

Japanese patients: fibrinogen levels in, 60; hypertrophic cardiomyopathy in, 112; incidence of coronary disease in, 40

kava, 210–11

khella: for angina, 70, 71; for lowering high blood pressure, 54, 56; for valvular heart disease, 126, 131

Klein, Alan, 229

L-arginine: for heart failure, 107, 119; for valvular heart disease, 136
L-carnitine, 188–89; for angina pectoris, 70, 71; for heart attacks, 98; for heart failure, 106–7, 119; for lowering cholesterol, 181; magnesium and, 184; for valvular heart disease, 131, 136
L-taurine, 56
lactose, 153
lasers, 73–74
LDL. *See* low density lipoproteins (LDL, "bad" cholesterol)
leaky valves, 121, 124
lectins, 161–62
left bundle branch block, 27
left heart failure, 104–5
left ventricle, 13–14
lesions, 35
Levinson, David, 57
licorice, 212–13
Lidocaine, 3, 142
lifestyle modifications: after having a heart attack, 97–98; lifestyle changes for lowering high blood pressure, 55
linolenic and linoleic fatty acids, 155, 192
Lipetz diet, 158–60
Lipetz, Phillip, 158
Lipid Research Clinic Coronary Primary Prevention Trial, 40–41
lipids, 34, 35; hypercholesterolemia and, 36; serum, 188–89, 228
lipoproteins, 39; LPa, 36, 46, 52–53, 178. *See also* high density lipoproteins (HDL); low density lipoproteins (LDL)
liquid herb extractions, 201
liquid oils, 155
lisinopril, 116–17
liver: cancer, 11; liver problems and statins, 47
low density lipoproteins (LDL, "bad" cholesterol), 39, 50–51; aerobic training and, 217; choles-terol-lowering medications, 45, 46, 47, 49; diabetes, 55–56; garlic in lowering, 204; gugulipid in lowering, 206–7; niacin in lowering, 178; oxidized LDL, 50
LPa (lipoprotein a), 36; in coronary artery disease, 39, 52–53; niacin and, 46, 178
lupus, 131
lysine, 157, 188
lysyl-oxidase, 186

McCulley, Kilmer, 60, 179
macrobiotic diet, 166
macromolecules, 152
macrophages, 34, 50
magnesium, 84, 170, 183–85; for heart attacks, 96–97, 99; for heart failure, 107, 119; L-carnitine and, 188; for lowering high blood pressure, 54, 56; for migraines, 212; for valvular heart disease, 128, 131, 136, 137
malnutrition, 111
mammary arteries, 76–77
manitol, 153
Master's two-step exam (stress test), 25
mechanical heart valves, 132, 133, 134, 135–36
medications: for angina pectoris, 65–70; cholesterol-lowering, 41, 42, 43–44, 45–50, 64; generic and trade name drugs, 271–74; for heart attacks, 89; for unstable angina, 82
meditation, 30
Mediterranean diet, 164
men: benign prostatic hypertrophy (BPH) in, 211, 212; coronary artery disease in, 35, 36, 37; idiopathic dilated cardiomyopathy in, 108, 110; mitral regurgitation in, 124; in observational studies, 40–42; popular diet for, 164–66; saw palmetto for, 211, 212
menopause: estrogen replacement

therapy, 48; women and coronary artery disease, 35–36
methionine, 157
metoprolol, 148
migraine headaches, 212
milrinone, 117
mindfulness-based stress reduction (MBSR), 231–34
minerals, 183–88
mitochondrial theory of heart failure, 106–7
mitral annular calcification (MAC), 125
mitral regurgitation, 124–28
mitral stenosis, 121–24
mitral valve annulus, 124–25
mitral valve prolapse (MVP), 127–28, 138, 189
mitral valve replacements, 124, 126
mitral valves, porcine, 135
mode, exercise, 216
monoclonal hypothesis, coronary artery disease and, 34
monocytes, 50
monosaccharides, 152–53
monounsaturated fats, 154, 155
mucilaginous herbs, 197, 199–200, 214
Multiple Risk Factor Intervention Trial (MRFIT), 40, 52, 58, 226
multivitamin/multimineral supplements, 7–8, 84, 137
murmurs, heart, 19, 22, 138
Murray, Michael T., 172, 211–12
myocardial infarctions. *See* heart attacks (myocardial infarctions)

naringin, 209
National Cholesterol Education Program (NCEP), 50–51, 52–53
National Heart, Lung, Blood Institute (NHLBI) Type 2 Coronary Intervention Study, 42
National Institutes of Health, 50
National Research Council, Food and Nutrition Board, 173–74
natural medicine, 2; natural meth-

ods of treating heart attack patients, 96–101; natural regimens for valvular heart disease, 136–37; natural remedies for aortic regurgitation, 131; natural remedies for chronic stable angina, 70; natural remedies for congestive heart failure, 119; natural remedies for heart failure, 106–7; natural remedies for unstable angina, 84; natural ways to keep hearts healthy, 7–8
Naturally Slim and Powerful (Lipetz), 158–59
neurally mediated syncope, 147–48
New Cabbage Soup Diet, The (Danbrodt), 166
niacin (nicotinic acid), 46, 177–78; for lowering cholesterol, 17, 42, 181; rhabdomyolysis, 48
Niaspan, 178
nifedipine, 68, 69, 131
Nihansan study, 40
nitrates, 65, 66, 68, 82, 92, 96
nitric oxide, 34, 66, 99
nitrogen, 157
nitroglycerine, 66, 68, 79, 89, 92, 96
nitrovasodilators, 115–16
No Flush Niacin, 178
nonatherosclerotic heart attacks, 88
noninvasive labs, 22
nuclear stress tests, 26–27, 28, 29
nutritive herbs, 197, 200, 214

obesity, 36, 38, 52, 57
oleic acid, 155
oligosaccharides, 153
omega-3 fatty acids (DHA and EPA), 154–55, 192–93; for angina pectoris, 71; for heart attacks, 98–99, 100; for heart failure, 107; for lowering cholesterol, 183; for lowering high blood pressure, 56; for lowering triglycerides, 52; for valvular heart disease, 136
omega-6 fatty acids, 155, 192, 193
omega-9 fatty acids, 155

onions, 56
oral estrogen therapy, 49
Ornish, Dean, 151
Ornish and Pritikin diet, 163–64
osteoporosis, 48
oxidative stressors, 175

pacemakers, 145, 184, 257–58
palpitations, heart, 21, 127, 184, 190, 258–59
panax ginseng, 182
pantethine, 43, 180, 181
papillary muscles, 125; papillary muscle rupture, 94
pectin, 47, 99, 100, 154
peppermint, 198, 214
peptic ulcer disease, 212–13
percutaneous transluminal coronary angioplasty (PTCA), 71, 72, 74
pericardium, 12, 23, 142
peripheral vascular disease, 20
Perloff's criteria, 127
phenols, 199
phenylalanine, 157
phosphatidyl choline, 180
phosphodiesterase inhibitors, 117–18
pig heart valves, 135
Pizzorno, Joe, 172
plaque, 18, 23, 26, 27; as cause for heart attacks, 88; lesions, 35
plasminogen activator inhibitor 1 (PAI-1), 47, 59
polysaccharides, 152, 153
polyunsaturated fats, 154, 155
porcine heterografts, 135
porcine valve replacement, 135
positron emission tomography (PET) scan, 28
post-herpetic neuralgia, 206
potassium, 54, 90, 170, 187
Pravastatin, 41
Pravastatin Limitation of Atherosclerosis in the Coronary Arteries Trial (PLAC 1), 44
pre-infarction angina, 80

premenstrual syndrome (PMS), 185
Prescription for Nutritional Healing (Balch and Balch), 167
Prilosec, 18
primary angioplasty, 90, 91
primary prevention trials, 40–41
Pritikin diet, Ornish and, 163–64
proanthocianidins, 207–8
procyanodolic oligomers, 207
progesterone, 49
programmed electrical stimulation (PES), 145
PROMISE Trial, 117
propranolol, 148
proprioceptive neuromuscular facilitation (PNF), 221, 222
Proscar, 212
prostaglandins, 168, 178
protein, 157–58
PROVED (clinical trial), 114
Prozac, 159
psychoneuroimmunology (PNI), 10, 227–28
psyllium, 47, 99, 100, 154
pulmonary autograft, 135
pulmonary edema, 104
pulmonic valve disease, 132
pulmonic valves, 131
Purkinje fibers, 16
Pygeum, 212
pyridoxine, 43, 179, 181

quercetin, 208–9

RADIANCE (clinical trial), 114
radio frequency (RF) ablation, 141, 262
raffinose, 153
Reapro, 75
Recommended Dietary Allowances (RDAs), 174
relaxation response, 230–31
Relaxation Response, The (Benson), 231
resistance training, 216, 218–20
response to injury hypothesis, coronary artery disease and, 34

rest images, stress images and, 26–27
restenosis, 72, 74, 75, 124
resting heart rate, 67
resting stress tests, 27–28
restrictive cardiomyopathy (RCM), 108, 109
rhabdomyolysis, 47–48
rheumatic heart disease, 123, 124, 131
rheumatoid arthritis, 123, 131
rhythm disturbances, heart. *See* heart rhythm disturbances
right ventricle, 13
rose hips fruit, 200, 214
Rosenman, Ray, 226
rotablator, 73
roughage, 153
Rubin, David, 139

St. Jude bioprosthetic valve, 133, 134
St. Thomas Atherosclerosis Regression Trial (STARS), 43–44
salicylate, 199
saponins, 199
sarsaparilla root, 199, 214
SAVE trial, 116
saw palmetto, 211, 212
Scandinavian Simvastatin Survival Study, 44
scurvy, 173
Sears, Barry, 164, 165
secondary prevention trials, 40, 42
sedentary stress tests, 27–28
selenium, 84, 170, 187–88
senile calcific aortic stenosis, 128
serotonin, 158–59, 160
serum lipids, 188–89, 228
Seven Country Study, 40
severe mitral stenosis, 123
silent ischemia, 64, 228
Simvastatin, 44
Sinatra, Steven, 189
single vessel disease, 71
sinoatrial node (S-A node), 15
slippery elm, 200, 214

smoking: as risk factor for coronary heart disease, 36, 38; tobacco, 53–54, 175; vitamin C and, 177
social isolation, 228
sorbitol, 153
soy, 182
spirulina algae, 200, 214
stachyose, 153
Starr-Edwards mechanical heart valve, 133
statins, 46, 47–48, 49, 191
stenosis/stenoses, 24
stents, 74, 75, 84
stress, 223–25; "fight or flight" response, 9, 105–6, 223; mindfulness-based stress reduction (MBSR), 231–34; our reactions to, 225–28; stress reduction techniques, 30, 97, 228–30; transcendental meditation and the relaxation response, 5, 7, 230–31
stress images, 26
stress tests, 2, 24–28
stretching, 221–22
strokes, 54
studies, observational: angioplasty, 71; aspirin, 64; atrial fibrillation, 265–66, 267; bypass surgery, 77–78; cholesterol-lowering, 40–45; coronary heart disease, 35–36, 49; exercise, 217; heart failure, 114, 116, 117; high blood pressure, 54; migraine headaches, 212; obesity, 57; omega-3 fatty acids, 52; smoking, 53; Type A behavior pattern, 58, 226; vitamin E, 176
subacute bacterial endocarditis (SBE), 137–38
sucrose, 153
sudden cardiac death, 30, 106, 112, 127
sugar alcohols, 153
superoxide dismutase, 172
supplements, natural: cholesterol-lowering, 17, 39, 42–43, 181–83; fiber, 57; for heart attack pa-

tients, 98–99; for lowering high blood pressure, 54, 56; omega-3 fatty acid supplements, 155; that help manage cardiac conditions, 190. *See also* vitamins

surgery: aortic stenosis, 130; coronary artery bypass grafting, 1, 4, 76–80; mechanical and prosthetic valves in valve replacement, 135–36; mitral valve, 123–24, 126–27

symptomatic mitral stenosis, 123

syncope, 112, 129, 147–48

systole, 13, 105, 124

systolic and diastolic dysfunction, 105

tachycardias, 168, 260–69

T'ai Chi Chuan, 23

tannins, 198

taurine, 99, 100, 184

Text Book of Internal Medicine (Harrison), 171

Textbook of Cardiology (Braunwald), 65

thiamine, 107, 111, 119, 174

threonine, 157

thrombolytics, 82, 87, 88, 90, 91

thrombus, 88

tinctures, 201

tissue valve replacements, 135

tobacco, 53–54, 175

torsade de pointes, 184

trans-fatty acids, 155–56

transcendental meditation and the relaxation response, 230–31

transcutaneous therapy, 49

transesophageal echocardiogram (TEE), 22–23

transient ischemic attacks (TIAs), 127

transient ventricular fibrillation, 129

transluminal extraction catheter (TEC), 72–73

transmyocardial revascularization (TMR), 80

transplants, heart, 118

treadmills, 25

tricuspid regurgitation (TR), 132

tricuspid stenosis (TS), 131–32

tricuspid valve, 13

tricuspid valve endocarditis, 132

triglycerides, 45, 47; aerobic training and, 217; beta blockers and, 67; dietary fat and, 154; elevated, 48, 49, 51–52; L-carnitine in lowering, 188–89; niacin in lowering, 178; vitamin C in lowering, 177

trimethylglycine, 98

tryptophan, 157, 159, 160, 177

tumeric, 47, 182

tumors, 23

Tylenol, 66

Type A behavior pattern, 36, 38, 58, 226

ultrafast (electron beam) CT, 28

ultrasounds, 22, 23

unopposed estrogen, 48–49

unstable angina, 80–85

VA Cooperative Study, 77–78

valerian, 198, 211, 214

valerotropes, 198

valine, 157

valvular heart disease, 121; abnormalities of the right heart valves, 131–32; aortic regurgitation, 130–31; aortic stenosis, 128–30; aortic valve disease, 128; cardiac valve prostheses, 132–36; mitral regurgitation, 124–28; mitral stenosis, 121–24; pulmonic valve disease, 132

vasconstriction, 106

vascular dilation, 66

vascular endothelial growth factor (VEG-F), 80

vasodilators, 69, 70, 131

vasospasm, 81

Vasotec, 115, 116

vasovagal syncope, 147

vegetable oils, 155

vein grafts, 76

ventricular fibrillation, 227, 266–69
ventricular septal defect (VSD), 94
ventricular systole, 13
verapamil, 69
very low density lipoproteins (VLDL), 39, 48, 52
VHeFT 2 Trial, 116
Viagra, 34, 66
vitamin A and the carotenoids, 175
vitamin B3, 42, 46
vitamin B6, 60, 98, 100, 169, 179
vitamin B12, 60, 98, 100, 169, 179–80
vitamin C, 43, 50, 59, 170, 172, 176–77; for angina pectoris, 70, 71; for bacterial endocarditis, 138; for heart attacks, 98, 99; for lowering cholesterol, 181; for unstable angina, 84
vitamin E, 43, 50, 59, 170, 172, 175–76; for angina pectoris, 70, 71; for anticoagulation, 134; essential fatty acids and, 193; for heart attacks, 98, 99; L-carnitine and, 188; magnesium and, 184; for unstable angina, 84
vitamins and minerals, 42–43, 171–73; food sources of important, 169–70; minerals, 183–88; nutritive herbs, 200; other helpful supplements, 188–89, 191–93; vitamins, 173–80

water with fiber supplements, 47
water-soluble fibers, and lower cholesterol, 39, 99, 100
weight training, 216, 218–20
West of Scotland Coronary Prevention Study, 41
Western Collaborative Group Study, 58, 226
wheat bran, 154
white willow bark, 199, 214
Willix, Robert, 237–38
Wolff-Parkinson-White (WPW) syndrome, 140–41, 262–63
women: bypass grafting in, 78–79; coronary artery disease in, 35–36, 37; estrogen replacement therapy, 48–50; mitral stenosis in, 124; PMS, 185; serotonin levels in, 158–59
World Health Organization Cooperative Trial, 41

xylitol, 153

ylang-ylang, 198, 214, 230
yoga, 30, 233

zinc, 186
Zocor, 84
Zone diet, 164–66